INSPIRE ME WELL

INSPIRE ME WELL

FINDING MOTIVATION TO TAKE CONTROL OF YOUR HEALTH

LISA BÉLANGER
WITH SARAH O'HARA

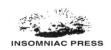

INSOMNIAC PRESS

Library and Archives Canada Cataloguing in Publication

Bélanger, Lisa, 1985-
Inspire me well : finding motivation to take control of
your health / Lisa Bélanger.

ISBN 978-1-55483-087-9

1. Health. 2. Lifestyles--Health aspects. I. Title.

RA776.B43 2012   613   C2012-905396-1

The publisher gratefully acknowledges the support of the
Department of Canadian Heritage through the Canada Book Fund.

Printed and bound in Canada

Insomniac Press
520 Princess Avenue, London, Ontario, Canada, N6B 2B8
www.insomniacpress.com

Canadä

Lisa Bélanger:

For all the cancer survivors I have worked with: you inspire me every day.

Sarah O'Hara:

To Paul O'Hara: the memory of your kind heart, passion for life, and love for family inspires me to live well every day.

Disclaimer

This book and related websites provide evidence-based nutritional and physical activity information in an educational manner only, and contains information that is general in nature and is not specific to the reader or any individual in particular. The contents of this book are intended to provide lifestyle information to aid in the personal wellness efforts of the reader.

The information in this book should not be interpreted as personal advice or medical diagnosis, and must not be used as such. Any information provided about chronic conditions or other ailments is general in nature; the publishers, authors, and any other parties involved in the writing or delivery of this book do not claim to be experts in any specific chronic condition. The information provided in this book does not cover all possible uses, actions, precautions, side effects, or interactions of medicines, dietary supplements, medical procedures, or lifestyle change. The information presented in this book should not be considered as complete and does not discuss all afflictions or treatments.

Always consult with your physician and other relevant registered health care professionals before beginning any physical activity, weight management, medication, dietary supplement, or health/wellness program. This book and its related websites should not be used to replace consultation with a registered health care professional. We strongly advise that the reader consult with a physician or other appropriate health care professional before adopting any of the suggestions in this book or before drawing any conclusions from its content.

No Warranties

The authors, publishers, and all other parties involved in the writing and publication of this book do not guarantee or warrant the quality, accuracy, completeness, timeliness, appropriateness, or suitability of the information presented in this book, nor of any product or services referenced by this book.

Acknowledgements

This book is a collaboration that would not have been possible without an incredible support team. We would like to jointly thank Gillian Buckley for her fantastic editing notes laced with the occasional humourous remark to lighten our moods during hectic days and nights of edits. A big thank you to Insomniac Press for providing us with the opportunity to complete an item that appears on both our Life Lists.

Thank you to those who provided interviews or information; special thank yous to Sheila Garland, Mélanie DesChâtelets, Michelle Emmerling, Linda Sparrowe, Vanessa Charlton, Dr. Nick Holt, Jessica Ferguson, and Craig Washka. Thank you to John Stanton for writing a thoughtful and kind foreword for this book and Tim Caulfield for contributing the afterthought; it is humbling to read such wonderful words about this project from people so influential in Canadian health.

To our families, friends, and colleagues who provided insight, feedback, and encouragement throughout this process: we couldn't have done it without you. Special thanks from Lisa: to Sarah for believing in my crazy ideas and stepping into this adventure with me, to Camilla Knight for providing information and humour throughout the writing process, to Kelley Keehn for my first introduction to the publishing process, and to Jane Knight for constantly providing me the confidence and persistence to go for my dreams. Special thanks from Sarah: to Lisa for being an enthusiastic partner-in-writing and friend, to Martin and Gloria Garnett for their love and support, to Libby and Megan O'Hara for their blessing and encouragement, and especially to Ryan O'Hara, my incredibly supportive husband, who graciously provided me with the patience, space, and encouragement to contribute to this book.

Finally, the heart of this book belongs to our contributors: thank you so much to Richard Bodnuruk, Ann MacDonald, Glori Meldrum, Martin Parnell, Crystal Phillips, Ashley Rose, and Judy Yawney for sharing your stories. Thank you also to Ed House and Sheldon Clark, whose names have been changed. You are all so very truly inspirational to us.

Contents

Foreword
By John Stanton

Inspire Me Well masterfully explores the correlation between exercise, eating well, and living a healthy life. You will find it to be an indispensible source of motivation, inspiration, and reflection.

Detailed inside are stories of people who have transformed their own lives and those of others by seeking out new levels of fitness and developing positive physical, nutritional, and mental habits. The book is filled with a plethora of science-based information, delivered using a practical and sensible approach. The focus is on your overall health and the things you can control in life each day.

The brilliant delivery isn't a quick fix, but rather encourages us to examine why our lives arrive at certain points and how, on assessment, we can achieve our life goals.

This book is packed with stories of real-life people who discovered the important factors of how to engage life-altering behavioural change. There is the story of the young mom, faced with her son's lymphoma, who discovered the value of social support and created an innovative way to give back to her community, while still providing a model of healthy behaviour for her own family. You will be equally inspired by the story of a former Canadian Forces soldier who put a stop to the cycle of obesity with his "can do" vision and his journey to learn the role of body composition in fitness.

While the chapters are filled with motivation and inspiration, they are also filled with practical and sensible ideas to implement change into your life. The stories encourage you to value health, nutrition, and exercise on a lifelong basis.

Learn the important illness risk factors and how the correlation between exercise and body weight can impact your life. Read the story of the cancer survivor whose life was saved with an understanding of the importance of taking care of both her body and her mind.

The reflections of real-life people overcoming great obstacles by changing their life patterns who then go on to influence others in the community will move you. You will be inspired when you read the story of Martin, who, at 47, committed to running 250 marathons in one year. Martin took on this challenge not just for the many physical and mental gifts it bestowed on him, but for his passion to support an international humanitarian organization, Right To Play.

A triple win theme is clearly evident in each success story. Not only do the contributors' healthy lifestyles benefit society as a whole by reducing health care costs, they have all experienced profound personal changes that have encouraged them to go on to help organizations and special groups.

Fit the profile of someone desiring change? You too can initiate change, like the subjects of the stories in this book, when given the knowledge, structure, and support by authors Sarah O'Hara and Lisa Bélanger. By sharing these stories with you, they hope to inspire similar shifts towards a healthy lifestyle in you, the reader.

Enjoy this riveting read, but more importantly, find fulfillment through a proactive approach to changing your lifestyle.

John Stanton is the CEO and founder of the Running Room, a member of the Order of Canada, and author of eight books on running and walking. He is a recipient of the Canadian Cardiovascular Society Dr. Harold N. Segall Award of Merit, an Honourary Doctor of Laws degree from the University of Alberta, and the Canadian Medical Association Award for Excellence in Health Promotion.

He has been inducted into the Canadian Retail Hall of Fame and the Alberta Business Hall of Fame and is the Hon. Lt. Col. of the Loyal Edmonton Regiment (4 PPCLI). He is a recipient of the Alberta Centennial Medal and the Queen's Diamond Jubilee Medal.

Stanton is regularly featured in the National Post, The Globe and Mail, *Vancouver's* The Province, *and other media across Canada. He has run over 60 marathons, hundreds of road races, and numerous triathlons, including the Hawaiian World Championship Ironman competition.*

Introduction

The Authors' Stories of Inspiration

Lisa's Inspiration

When I'm asked what motivates me to be active, to eat well, and to live a healthy life, I can pinpoint the answer to one brief phone call that I will never forget. My friend Jane and I had plans one night, and when it came time to get together I could not get hold of her. I was frustrated and slightly hurt that she blew me off, so I went over to my then-boyfriend's house. While we were watching basketball, the phone rang. I was surprised it was for me—it was Jane. She was at the hospital waiting for test results she had done earlier that day. She felt so guilty for breaking our plans that she called my house for my boyfriend's number. She said, "They think I have cancer, and when I heard that, all I wanted to do was talk to you." The summer between Grade 11 and senior year, my best friend Jane was diagnosed with Hodgkin's lymphoma.

That phone call, those few seconds, changed my life more than I could have ever imagined. At 17, I watched my best friend have more needles poked in her, more drugs injected into her than the average person does in a lifetime, and I watched her fight for her life. She lost her hair but never lost her beautiful smile. After a gruelling two-year battle, she passed away. I will never forget holding her hand while she gasped for air and was drugged so that she could not feel the pain while I said goodbye.

Your perception of life changes when you are staring at death. Jane and I created a "bucket list" of things we wanted to accomplish before we died. It is now up to me to work through the list. This list has allowed me to live life to a depth I could never have even imagined. Every day, every breath is a treasure. Although I miss Jane and selfishly I want her with me, I know she inspires me every day.

When Jane was alive, she said: "You only get one body, and it is your temple." I realized then how much we take our health for granted. I realized that when I woke up I just expected my body to function without continuously working at it and fuelling it properly. This shifted my perspective on my own health. There are behaviours I can control to improve my physical and mental health that will allow me to do everything I want in life and to be able to check off everything on that bucket list.

I have the honour and privilege to work with cancer patients and survivors every day. These people have the most incredible perspective on life. This life, your health, is a gift. This "aha" moment should happen many years before someone becomes sick. This thought is what inspired this book.

At a young age I got to question my own mortality, and for that I have to say I am thankful. It allows me to truly live. It has inspired me to bungee jump, travel, pursue my PhD, and to challenge myself at every opportunity. I had always enjoyed physical activity, but now it is more than a game; it allows me to do the things I want, makes me feel better every day, and I know I am doing what I can for my health.

Lisa Bélanger, MSc, CSEP-CEP

Sarah's Inspiration

As a generally healthy kid, I had never given much thought to the importance of physical activity and healthy eating—that was always my parents' job. I guess you could say I was lucky: I grew up in a household where activity was encouraged but not forced, and home-cooked healthy meals were the norm. I always had a healthy body weight and a great social network. The same could be said for my husband, whose natural athleticism kept him busy year-round and whose parents valued the benefits of feeding good food to their two children. It wasn't until we reached university that I really began to grasp the potential harm that could come from the absence of a healthy lifestyle.

In 2005, my husband's father was diagnosed with colon cancer at age 50. Despite the family history of cancer, the diagnosis was a shocking blow to both his family and mine. With a strong academic background in the sciences, I knew that genetic susceptibility can play a role in many chronic diseases such as cancer. I also had learned, however, that environment can play an equally or more important role in the risk of disease. When I considered that my father-in-law, like so many Canadian adults, had once been an extremely active and healthy young man who gradually became less active and more overweight with age, I couldn't help but wonder whether the development or progression of his cancer could have been slowed or counteracted by maintaining a healthier lifestyle.

Following his initial success with chemotherapy treatment and a period of remission, we received news in the summer of 2007 that his cancer had returned. This news was somehow even more devastating than the initial diagnosis; over the following weeks and months his condition declined, and eventually we would learn that the cancer had spread to his liver and abdomen. We lost Paul in the early hours of New Year's Day 2008. To see my husband's family lose him, and to see his own father outlive him, was more than I could accept. It wasn't long after the funeral that I made a personal vow to commit myself to a career of health promotion and the prevention and management of chronic disease.

I truly believe that my father-in-law's death was not in vain; my mother-in-law is now an active volunteer for early cancer advocacy, and his children are healthier than they've ever been—they, as I, have come to realize the importance of good health and preventative living. Paul's memory, for me, serves as a daily reminder of the importance of achieving and maintaining a healthy lifestyle of homemade meals, regular exercise, and relaxation for stress relief. Although genetics can play a role in the risk for chronic disease, it is often a less-than-healthy lifestyle that exacerbates this risk. As a Registered Dietitian, I have clients who are fighting for their health inspiring me on a daily basis. I have seen clients able to reduce or eliminate their need for certain medications by improving their lifestyles. I don't claim to be perfect, but I try to carefully weigh the decision to deviate from a lifestyle that I know will give me the best chance at a long and healthy life. If the forces of nature are against me and I do develop illness or disease in my lifetime, I want to know that my daily decisions were ones that ensured I was doing everything within my power to stay healthy. We each get only one body and one life, and good health gives us the freedom to enjoy it to the fullest. I hope this book encourages each reader, whether relatively healthy or battling illness/disease, to realize the incredible effects of positive thinking and living well.

Sarah O'Hara, RD

Chapter 1

An Introduction to the Journey Known as Health

"He who cures a disease may be the skillfullest, but he that prevents it is the safest physician." — Thomas Fuller

Some people make healthy food choices, make sure to sweat at least once daily through physical activity, and place significant value in their health and well-being. You know the ones: when you look at them you wonder where they find the time and get the energy. The majority of us, however, do not have this mindset.

We have become a society that relies on convenience food and overloads on fat, sugar, and salt. Food is starting to be less like food and more like plastic and engineered to last longer, look better, and cost less with little regard to the health content or the negative effect the product or packaging has on our bodies. Most of the food we eat today our grandparents would not even recognize as food. We tend to microwave, order in, and go out to restaurants more than ever. Consequently we know less and less about what is in our food. The majority of us have absolutely no idea what we are putting into our bodies.

Recently I saw a public awareness commercial against childhood obesity that showed a young boy, probably about four or five, colouring at a table. A woman (presumably his mother) comes in and sits down at the table with him. She has a brown paper lunch bag, and from this bag she pulls out drugs and a syringe. The woman starts preparing the drugs for injection by heating them and putting them in the syringe. She then ties the boys arm as if to inject him. Just as you think she is going to insert the needle into the boy's arm, she hands him a fast-food hamburger. Text comes up that reads: "You wouldn't inject your child with junk, so why are we feeding it to them?" (You can view this video on YouTube, it is called "Breaking the Habit—Childhood Obesity Ad Australia.")

This video gave me chills the first time I saw it. I thought it did a brilliant job to illustrate the point that what we ingest is critical. It goes back to the old saying "You are what you eat." Unfortunately, poor eating has become such a norm that we tend not to think about how ingesting junk can turn our bodies to junk. This thought is also relevant, as the video portrays, to what we are feeding the next generation.

In addition to developing poor eating habits, we spend the majority of our time sitting or lying down. Technology is making it easier and easier for us to move less. It seems as though the more evidence there is of the catastrophic effect of these poor habits, the worse we get. As humans, we need to move daily. It is how we are built. As you read on in this book, you will see how extremely important this is. Then why is physical education being cut from our schools? Why aren't there more campaigns out there to get us moving? I assure you, it is a source of great frustration for me that we need obesity to get to epidemic proportions before we will begin to see the errors of our ways.

We are eating more and moving less than ever. Knowing that these behaviours are directly linked to an increased risk for chronic diseases (cancer, heart disease, diabetes, kidney failure, anxiety, and many more), do we have the power (or yet, the willpower) to reverse this trend? Can we start teaching and inspiring behaviours that will aid in negating this epidemic of sedentary behaviour?

The world seems to be moving at an increasingly quicker pace, forcing many of us to leave our health behind. As stress levels increase, sleep decreases. Televisions, computers, and smart phone screens also influence our sleep patterns. Many problems that concern this generation didn't even exist to the same extent in past generations.

I read a quotation the other day that said: "The best time to plant a tree was 20 years ago; the second best time is now." It is never too late to change your daily health habits. The instant you start, you will begin to see and experience the benefits of your actions.

As in life, there are many aspects of our health that we are not able to control. There is not much we can do about our genetics, some aspects of environmental exposure, age, race, and ethnicity. There are, however, many risk factors that we know we can modify, such as exercise, nutrition, sleep, stress levels, sex practices, other environmental exposures, smoking, blood pressure, wearing a seat belt, and sun exposure. Throughout this book we will be discussing what I like to call the "Big Four." The Big Four are the health behaviours that have the most influence on your life and can directly or indirectly affect the other health behaviours. Beyond that, making changes in one area of the Big Four will most likely create changes in the other three health behaviours. The areas are exercise, nutrition, sleep, and stress.

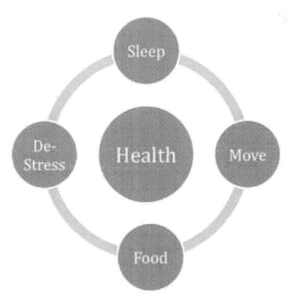

As you can see from the graph, the Big Four are strongly linked. For example, studies have shown that if you start a daily exercise routine (provided it is not too close to your bedtime), you will dramatically improve your sleep length and quality. Conversely, if you are getting enough high-quality sleep, you may be more apt to have the energy for your daily workouts.

A second example would be that proper nutrition helps to ensure your energy levels are well-regulated throughout the day, which improves productivity in all of your daily activities. Feeling energized is also important when it comes to physical activity. Properly fuelling your body for activity will lead to better results and improved stamina, whether your goal is to run a marathon or to be able to go ice skating with your kids.

Another example would be that if you are effectively managing your stress, you will be less likely to overeat or emotionally eat. Research shows that under stressful situations, we eat more calories. Over time this may lead to weight gain and increased physical and psychological stress. We are also more likely to reach for comfort or convenience foods that are high in fat, sugar, and/or salt during stressful times, which promote this same vicious cycle of overeating.[1]

I have the privilege to work every day with cancer patients and survivors at the cancer-only fitness centre where I work and do my research. As much as possible we try to work with them one on one. The cancer fitness centre is a unique facility that has no TVs, and social interactions with staff and other participants are strongly encouraged.

The survivors are a constant reminder to live in the "now." When cancer survivors come into the fitness centre to work with me, I get to know them very well. A conversation that I often have with participants is how their cancer has turned into a "teachable moment" to really put perspective on their lives. They say things such as, "Now I will start and continue an exercise regime," "Now I will start eating well," "Now I will quit that extremely stressful job I do not enjoy." I completely understand how an illness can be the kick in the pants needed to realize that changes need to be made. My hope in writing this book is that we can inspire that "aha" moment and encourage lifestyle changes *before* you are affected by illness. No matter what your age, what you do now, today, for your health can dramatically affect your future.

What inspires people to live well? What motivates them to take care of their bodies, their vessels? Is it simply to prolong their expiration date or is there something more? Researchers have explored these very complex behaviours for centuries. The benefits of healthy eating and physical activity are countless—there is no debate there. The problem is the disconnect between knowledge and behaviour; researchers tend to look at these problems using behaviour change theories. Many of these theories include environmental influence, belief systems, norms, and intentions, among others. We propose a dash of inspiration.

To be inspired is a powerful means of action; when a situation inspires us to act, it is as though new life has been breathed into our souls and gives us purpose and meaning. Finding inspiration from others or from within ourselves can motivate us to complete even the most seemingly insurmountable of tasks.

This book will take an in-depth look at the inspiration behind behaviour using stories of people who make daily choices to promote their own health and well-being. Each story provides a glimpse into the lives of individuals who are inspired to prioritize their health and wellness. Through these stories, we can learn how to find or create inspiration from difficult situations and how to overcome the many barriers to optimal health. Many stories will come from individuals who have undergone life-changing events, for example cancer, that put their health into perspective.

Interspersed between the stories will be tips, ideas, and suggestions from a physical activity/behaviour change expert (Lisa) and a registered dietitian (Sarah). Content will be derived from the latest research, our extensive education on the topics, and on personal experiences within our respective industries. The goal is to provoke thought and to provide you with practical and easy ideas for action.

References

1. Born, JM et al. Acute Stress and Food-Related Reward Activation in the Brain During Food Choice During Eating in the Absence of Hunger. *Int J Obes* (Lond). 2010 Jan; 34(1): 172-81. Available online at: www.ncbi.nlm.nih.gov/pubmed/19844211

Chapter 2

Food for Thought

"We are what we repeatedly do. Excellence, then, is not an act, but a habit." — Aristotle

Our health is the sum of many small choices we make daily. Thinking about changing a behaviour or accomplishing a goal can be overwhelming. Start by analyzing your recent actions, choice by choice. For example: Do you purchase the chocolate bar or the pack of almonds at the convenience store? Will you take the bus or walk the 20 minutes to work today? At a wedding, will you sit it out or dance?

On the drive to a ball hockey game, I asked my friends (two twentysomething guys) what motivates them to complete their gym workouts. They came up with a variety of answers, such as performance in sports, physique, and, in last place, health. They followed up their reasons immediately with a "But *man* is it ever hard to get there sometimes." Many healthy behaviours do not necessarily provide the immediate pleasure that unhealthy behaviours do, but they have many long-term benefits. This is where motivation, willpower, social support, and creativity come into play.

Even though I know so much about the benefits of healthy eating and exercise, I completely understand these thoughts. I find it hard to get up, get out, and get to it. Here is an example:

One week I had made the plan to bike for 20 minutes every morning in order to start my day off on the right foot. Not only would it guarantee I got in the majority of my recommended physical activity minutes (the Canadian Physical Activity Guide recommends 150 minutes of moderate physical activity per week), but I decided that it would be a great addition to my current activity plan because it would strengthen the muscles around my injured knee.

One night I stayed up late playing ball hockey. When the alarm went off the next morning, I wanted to stay in bed more than I can express in words. While I realize that the devil and angel on the shoulders in cartoons are just a metaphor for your willpower, I swear this happened:

Angel: Time to start a new day.

Devil: Stay in bed; you need your sleep.

Angel: Biking will make you feel better all day, protect your knee from injury, and you'll earn a pat on the back for accomplishing your goal.

Devil: You are active enough. What is one day of sleeping in?

Angel: Get your sorry butt up and bike. *You* made the goal to bike and *you* are the only one who will reap benefits. (My angel is slightly aggressive.)

I am happy to say the angel won. But these are the small choices I am referring too. Even though it was "just one morning" as the devil so kindly pointed out, it is the small choices that create a habit. Those habits become who you are. With both activity and food choices, it takes making a specific choice day after day for at least three to four weeks in order for the behaviour to become a habit.

That morning, I got up, onto my bike and did my 20-minute ride. After only about five minutes of riding I felt better. After my 20 minutes of riding and a couple of stretches, I felt energized and was so happy I made the decision to follow through on my plans.

My friends said that once they do get out, they feel so good and even better after. I am sure this feeling comes from both the exercise itself and the knowledge that you beat the devil on your shoulder. You accomplished your goal and did something great for your body. That feeling is your body giving you a high-five for a job well done.

My point is that health is a journey—a never-ending one. It is the small choices you make every day that matter. I think this is what many people miss when they think about health. What is so exciting is that it means that your health, or at least the parts that you can modify, is under *your* control.

How people make these small choices is a question that researchers have been asking for years. What influences our decisions? Is it environment? People around us? Our beliefs? Our knowledge? Our inspirations? Our skill and abilities?

The answer is: all of the above.

We are going to suggest ways to improve your exercise, nutrition, and other aspects of health and wellness throughout this book, but even more importantly, as you work through this book, you should try to start to think of your own ideas. How can you make healthy choices every day and have fun doing it?

There are many theories about how health behaviours are formed; however, most rely on one central concept. Some theories call it self-efficacy, others call it perceived behavioural control. No matter what it's called, it is defined as the confidence someone has in performing a behaviour and how much control they have over the opportunity to perform it.

This form of behavioural change can be accomplished in a few different ways. The ones most traditionally studied are self-mastery experiences or reciprocal-mastery experiences. Self-mastery experiences are instances when you accomplish the desired behaviour. Reciprocal-mastery experiences are when you see or hear about a person similar to you who you can relate to accomplishing a desired behaviour.

Here is an example of a self-mastery experience: Your goal or desired behaviour change is to wake up every morning at 6 am and ride your stationary bike for 20 minutes. Every time you wake up at 6 am and ride the bike, you have more confidence that you can do this behaviour. With more confidence that you can do the behaviour, the more likely you will actually do it.

If your goal is to start playing tennis (a personal goal of mine) but have never played it before, it can be pretty intimidating standing all alone on your side of the court while balls are flying at you. To get onto the court, plan to go with a friend or book a lesson with a pro. If you are able to go out once, make that first step and get out there, you will be more confident that you can do it a second time. Then, after a second time, you will be more confident you can do it a third or fourth time.

Here is an example of a reciprocal-mastery experience: You're a 32-year-old woman who recently gave birth and you are thinking about running a 10K race. You have never run a race before and are not sure this is a reasonable goal. If you hear about another thirtysomething woman who just had a baby and has completed a 10K, you may consider this more reasonable. If you found out that all of the women in your Mommy and Me exercise group are also running a 10K, you may think this is even more possible.

Seeking out opportunities for reciprocal experiences will make you more likely to feel like you can accomplish a behaviour and more likely to try it. How do you seek out opportunities for reciprocal-mastery experiences? Start by dreaming and creating a goal, even if it is outside your comfort zone. Start discussing your goal with friends and family members. You may be surprised who may know someone who has a similar goal or who has been through it before. Another option is to search local facilities, newspapers, and online for a group with similar goals. In the example above, it would be a Mommy and Me exercise class. Another example would be someone who has never tried CrossFit. It can be intimidating the first few times; it is intense and has movements that may be unfamiliar. You may think that it is beyond your physical ability, until your friend who is of a similar fitness level is going regularly to classes and lifting more weight then you thought possible. This knowledge will increase the confidence in yourself that you can do it.

Some behavioural change theories talk about normative beliefs. How many important people in your life do, or support, the behaviour in question? For example, if you decided to start a walking program, who in your life already walks? And who in your life would—if you asked them—think your starting a walking program would be a good idea? If your best friends are already in a walking program and your spouse thinks that your starting a walking program is a good idea, you will be more likely to start a walking program than if you did not have the support. Social support will be examined in greater depth in Chapter 3.

I believe that if a behaviour is not enjoyable you just won't do it. The research strongly supports me on this one. When it comes to health behaviours, especially ones you do not innately enjoy, it is a matter of adding a bit of spice to make them fun. My supervisor often uses the example of broccoli. Very few people enjoy raw broccoli (I am one of those people, but that's beside the point), and even if you do, it tastes a little better by adding ranch dressing. This is the same for exercise. Very few people enjoy running on a treadmill in a dark basement. The actual physiological experience of exercise is not enjoyable: your heart racing, breathing heavy, muscles screaming, sweating…it just isn't pleasant. We prefer our exercise with "dip" by adding socializing, music, sport/competition, TV, etc. We literally trick our bodies into exercise by making it more appealing. This is key: If you want to make a behavioural change, you'll want to find something about this behaviour that you enjoy or find a way to make it enjoyable.

If you really do not like eating vegetables but know how beneficial they can be, you will be more likely to include them in your diet. You know that vegetables are a great source of nutrients, are full of bowel-friendly fibre, and are associated with reduced risk for illness and a variety of chronic conditions such as heart disease and certain cancers, and so you make the decision that the benefits outweigh the taste. The key to this, of course, is knowledge and understanding of the specific benefits and a personal connection with these benefits.

Your environment has a dramatic influence on your behaviour. For example, you are more likely to walk to the store if there are sidewalks—you'll feel safer and enjoy a more attractive walk. Another example is you are more likely to ride your stationary bike (or treadmill) if the area is attractive. The area should be well lit and provide something enjoyable to look at (I suggest a TV). Essentially, if you store your bike in the unfinished basement with nothing around, you are much less likely to use it.

There are some other things you can do to your environment that can help encourage you to change your behaviour. You can use prompts around your house, such as a sticky note to remind you to floss or placing *Canada's Food Guide* on the fridge. If you would like to do a morning run, try laying out your running clothes and running shoes the night before in a place where you can see them as soon as you wake up.

These prompts make the day-to-day decisions slightly easier. They remind you of the healthy behaviour you would like to perform, at the right opportunity. For behaviour change, you need to have both motive and opportunity. (Note: The same principles apply to murder one—not to be confused.)

In the following chapters, we will expand on these concepts and others that influence our health and our family's health and what that can mean in our daily lives. We have provided activities and more in-depth information on *www.inspiremewell.com*. If any of the specific topics interest you, be sure to check out the resources provided on the site.

Chapter 3

The Power of Support

"Participating in these charity endurance events has not only had an enormous impact on my physical and mental wellbeing, but has also changed the lives of my family (and extended family) members." — Ann MacDonald

We rarely need to examine our own strength, determination, and resilience. We do not know how strong we are until we have to be. Thinking of a loved one being diagnosed with a disease that is slowly taking their life is a nightmare. To live and breathe this for months, or years, as they go through treatments all the while feeling powerless is something that will shake you to your core. It forces you to ask: What is health? What do I have control over? Ann MacDonald is someone who embraces health and family after being faced with every parent's greatest fear. In doing so, she has set a tremendous example for her children, her husband, and her community. Following Ann's story, we will discuss the importance and influence of social support in health behaviours, as well as how parental support and sport can positively impact a child's view of physical activity for a lifetime.

Ann's Story: 5 for 5

My story began on May 4, 2005, when my son Parker was diagnosed with lymphoblastic lymphoma, a type of blood cancer. He was five years old at the time. Parker endured nine months of chemotherapy at Children's Hospital. He was always brave, kind, and tolerant of what he had to go through. His cancer experience has changed the way I look at life and the challenges it presents.

People sometimes ask me how I got through this difficult chapter of my life. First and foremost, I had incredible support from my family and friends. We also had an amazing patient in Parker. It was in 2006 that my family and I became involved with the Leukemia & Lymphoma Society and participated in their Light the Night Walk. In 2007, my sisters and I joined the society's Team in Training program. At that time, I had no idea of the impact that this organization would have on my family and me. In a relatively short time, the program transformed three ordinary moms into triathletes and cancer advocates. I can assure you, this was no small task. When we signed up, none of us had a bike, two of us had never run a mile, and two of us couldn't swim more than the length of a pool. I was in all three of these categories. People often think that because I'm thin that I've always been an athlete. But the truth is I haven't. As a matter of fact, I was one of the few children in elementary school not to get the Presidential Physical Fitness Award patch. If someone like me can change my fitness level so drastically, anyone can.

The first time I crossed the finish line was amazing. It was the St. Anthony's Triathlon in 2007. I remember seeing my teammates, my husband Bill, my sisters Mary and Elizabeth, and my mom. I cried tears of joy and relief that I had finished, and tears of sadness for Parker's cancer experience. It was one of the most emotional experiences of my life. One very touching moment of that finish was when a teammate said to me, "Some day you and Parker will cross the finish line together." At that time we were still very uncertain of Parker's health, and thinking of the future was emotionally risky but comforting. Participating in Team in Training has given me hope for the future, hope for a cure, and hope that some day Parker and I will cross that finish line together.

In February of 2011, Parker had his five-year checkup. I am

happy to let you know that all the news was good: no signs of cancer and no long-term damage from his chemotherapy. Today he is a healthy, happy, 12-year-old little boy. Five years earlier, I had said that when this day came, we would have a big party. So we did. Yet, while a party was appropriate, it didn't seem adequate. Even though the treatment saved Parker's life, it was a gruelling process, and he now has a 50 percent higher risk of developing cancer later in life due to exposure to radiation and chemotherapy. We won the battle to save his life; now we are fighting for his future. We have also lost friends along this journey. So I decided to do something special to celebrate Parker's survival and also honour the friends we've lost. That's when the "5 for 5" idea was born.

I was planning the big "5 for 5" in my mind and decided to send my sisters, Mary and Elizabeth, a text message about my dream of the three of us crossing the finish line of the Nike Women's Marathon together just as we had begun our journey in 2007—together! Their responses were "Are you drinking?" and "Put the wine down." (They know me too well.) Yet that crazy dream became a reality, and on October 16, 2011, the three of us crossed the finish line together in a celebration of survival and hope. I made the commitment to do five big endurance events in one year while raising money for cancer research. With my family's support, I completed a half marathon, two full marathons, and two century (100 mile) bike rides. We also raised over $21,000.

Since our first year in 2007, I have completed two half marathons, three full marathons, three Olympic-distance triathlons, and three century rides. My family has also raised around $75,000 for cancer research.

Participating in these charity endurance events has not only had an enormous impact on my physical and mental well-being, but has also changed the lives of my family (and extended family) members. My four children now participate in 5Ks, my husband is an avid cyclist and triathlete, and my siblings and their children are also physically active. We have also dramatically changed what we think is possible. Before Parker's cancer, if someone had told me that I would some day ride a bicycle 100 miles in one day or run a full marathon, I would have told them they were crazy. I know most people think the same way about themselves. I now have the gift of believing in new possibilities. I would encourage anyone who is considering signing up for an endurance event to do so with a charity. Not only will you be improving you own life, but you will also be changing the lives of others. I can guarantee that if you put in the work and dedication, your life will never be the same.

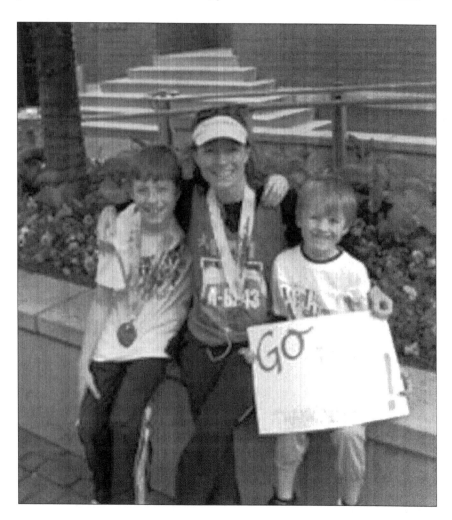

Social Support

Social support is defined as reassurance that one is cared for by and has assistance available from other people, and that one is part of a social network. The research behind social support and physical activity (or any health behaviour for that matter) is endless. Regardless of your age, gender, race/ethnicity, marital status, physical activity background, or income and education level, social support can positively affect your attendance and adherence to physical activity.

One of the main factors influencing whether or not you will be able to change a behaviour or accomplish a goal is having social support. Someone can provide social support in many different ways. People often think that the best way to support others is to participate in the desired behaviour with them or "go along for the run" like in Ann's story. This is a very powerful way to provide social support.

Another way to provide social support without actually participating in the behaviour is encouraging it. The great thing about encouragement is that it can be provided from a distance, over the phone, online, etc. Although Ann does not go into detail about it in her story, she received a huge amount of encouragement from friends, family, and people she did not know who provided donations and words of support. These can be great motivators. While Ann was out on her long runs, wondering if she should just slip away and take a cab the rest of the way, she thought of her son and all the people behind her and continued with her run.

Going one step further, you can support someone by giving them the opportunity to perform the behaviour. For example, if your spouse's goal is to get in a 30-minute walk every day, you could offer to do the dishes after dinner, giving him or her the opportunity to go for a walk. Another example: If you know your friend is trying to lose weight and eat healthily, instead of meeting for a beer, meet for a walk or choose a restaurant with healthy options. These small considerations can go a long way and are more meaningful than words of encouragement alone.

When you are planning a behavioural change, consider your support network. How can you get them involved? The first step is to tell them your goals and explain why you would like to accomplish the goals. It may surprise you where your support comes from and in what form.

Like Ann, you can also seek out social support outside of your current network. Say you would like to run your first half marathon. This is a lofty goal, and you would definitely benefit from going for runs with others. No one in your current social support network runs and you cannot convince them to start? (Ann lucked out being able to drag her sisters along.) Joining a local running club could be exactly what you need. It is a great way to learn proper running techniques, get helpful hints from experienced runners, meet new people, and, most importantly, have like-minded people working with you to accomplish your goal. As Meghan Kennedy said in her guest blog on *inspiremewell.com,* there is nothing more satisfying than a high-five from a running partner after a long hard run.

As mentioned above, social support is one of the keys to success for *all* health behaviours. This also includes healthy eating habits. As an example, take the family meal. Research shows that families who eat together eat healthier. Use the family meal, from the planning phase to the after-dinner cleanup, as an opportunity to teach your children healthy eating practices. Children are more likely to take an interest in eating well if they are involved in all aspects of the family meal (appropriate to age, of course). For example, the whole family can suggest meal ideas and help to make a grocery list for the week. Younger children can also help in the preparation of meals or snacks by helping to wash vegetables or fruit, and older children can begin to grate or chop with supervision and can also help with setting the table. The family meal provides an opportunity for parents to model healthy eating habits, such as eating all food groups on the plate (both familiar and new). It also provides invaluable bonding time with family members.

Another time when social support is helpful is when one family member is looking to make dietary changes, whether for weight loss, medical reasons (such as diabetes or kidney disease), or general wellness. If the entire family is not accepting and committed to the change, it can be an extremely difficult transition that is destined for failure. Providing support is so much more than simply saying, "I'll support you." It might also involve helping to search for new recipes, avoiding purchasing household foods that could sabotage the family member's efforts to eat well, or suggesting changing the usual weekly take-out pizza night to a healthier alternative.

As humans, we tend to be very social creatures and enjoy having shared experiences. Technology has only enhanced this with networks such as Facebook, LinkedIn, Twitter, and communication tools such as Skype. These are all tools to bring us closer together in our desire to share experiences. No matter what your goal, you will get greater results if you acquire social support, and you may be surprised by who you inspire.

Parental Influence

If you are a frequent flyer, I am sure you can say, word-for-word, the safety demonstration given prior to the airplane's takeoff. You know how they always say "If you are travelling with small children, put your oxygen mask on before your child's"? This is true of all health behaviours.

Parents influence their children's involvement in physical activity and sport in many different ways. It begins with the parent's own beliefs and health behaviours.

When I was reading through Ann's story, I wondered, how much do parents influence the activities of their children? Some of it is apparent; younger children are completely dependent on their parents for finances, enrollment, transportation, etc. But what makes children continue after they no longer need their parents in order to participate? How much influence do parents have on their children's thoughts and attitudes towards continuing to be active as they age?

Parents can be role models, interpreters, and providers of exercise. Parents who engage in physical activity or play sports on any level provide a model for their children and help normalize the activity. Albert Bandura, the "godfather of behaviourism," suggested that the underlying mechanisms of a child's learning are that the child internalizes the attitudes and behaviours of the role model.[1] Parents do not necessarily have to be competitive athletes; they could play recreationally, coach, officiate, or even be avid gym-goers. By participating in an activity, they demonstrate that physical activity is an appropriate behaviour. Basically, active parents have active children.

I coached soccer for several teams, from recreational soccer for both children and adults to competitive and high-school teams. When there were games or practices, parents would come to support their children and watch the games. Many of these parents were overweight. They would often bring their lawn chairs and sit while they watched their children being active. This never occurred to me to be an odd practice until I saw one of the fathers walking around the field as the players warmed up. Then I thought about it. Players at the more competitive levels were expected to be there 45 minutes before the game. Most parents stayed on site, sat down, and chatted. This father was taking that time to get his exercise in. BRILLIANT! He had already committed the time to be at the field, why not use it wisely? Not only was he getting his exercise in, he was doing it in plain view for the children to see.

Parents can act as interpreters of an experience; their beliefs and values communicate a subtle message to their children about physical activity. For example, do parents value and reward winning or effort when their children are engaging in sport? Excessive pressure to perform is related to negative consequences for the child (anxiety, burnout) while lower or moderate pressure on performance will promote children's enjoyment in physical activity. Having parents who value, enjoy, and compete in physical activity can increase the values, enjoyment, and competence that a child feels in physical activity compared with those children whose parents who do not value activity.[2]

Parents can encourage physical activity in many different ways; this goal can be accomplished by watching, coaching, and driving their children as they play in team sports. It can also come in the form of a monetary investment. There is no doubt that parental encouragement is directly related to children's participation in physical activity.

Reading through the literature in this area, I could not help but reflect on my own childhood, my parents, and their influence on my physical activity. It even lead to my studying and getting a doctorate in the subject. I remember learning in my first year of the Human Kinetics (Kinesiology) program at St. Francis Xavier University that over 70 percent of people are inactive and that there is an obesity epidemic. Where had I been? How had I missed it?

My sister was active, my friends were active, and I spent most of my younger years in a rink, at a field, or in a gym. However, in order for that to be the case, it started at home with my parents. As I learned about how inactive most people are, I called up my parents to thank them. There is no doubt in mind that they are the reason I was so active growing up. They also inspired a passion of lifelong learning on the topic.

Parents create what their children view as "normal." Consider this: I had an intriguing conversation with Camilla Knight, a recent PhD graduate whose research focuses on parental influence on children's sport participation. For one of her studies she interviewed children and asked them what they thought of their parents' play— do their parents play? The children's responses were eye-opening.

They said their parents used the word *play* to get them to leave, as in "go upstairs and play; I have to do my taxes." When they were asked specifically if their parents played, they said, "Yes, but it always seems so angry and boring." For example, one child described how his parents would sit around and watch Ultimate Fighting challenges on television. The adults would sit, watch, eat, and scream at the television. You can understand from children's eyes that this does not seem like fun at all.

The Influence of Sport

Sport can have an interesting influence on how we perceive physical activity. Although I truly believe sport is an incredible way to achieve the physical benefits of exercise and add enjoyment to exercise, it also teaches life skills, such as team building, resilience, and how to handle both success and failure. How sport is presented to a child can have a lasting influence.

Growing up, one of my best friends was a very competitive hockey player. He was on numerous elite teams, and if he was not at the rink for games or practices, he was playing outside with his friends. It was such a part of who he was. He lived and breathed hockey, as many young men do.

When he grew up, well...he didn't. He was short and not very big. His lack of height and stature stopped his competitive hockey career after high school. We went to different undergraduate universities but ended up in the same city after school. I kept nagging him to go play hockey or play in a ball hockey league. He would always say no. I was so confused; hockey was who he was. Sometime during his years of play he became unable to play ball hockey for enjoyment. If it was not competitive, he did not want to play. If he could not play to his high standards, he did not want to play.

He was once an elite athlete and now does very little activity outside of his manual labour job.

Another one of my friends growing up was my polar opposite.

While my life revolved around whatever sport season it was, she was into drama, on the student council, and had little to no interest in sport. When I would talk about the NHL, she would start singing a song in her head and pretend to listen. She did, however, participate in our physical education class right until Grade 12.

We also went to different undergraduate universities and lost touch. I kept tabs on her, of course, via Facebook and noticed she had gained a significant amount of weight. Five years after I had last seen her, I travelled to where she was living and connected with her for dinner. When she walked into the restaurant I was shocked. (I am sure I did a wonderful job at hiding my emotions.) She was stunning and about half the size of the girl I had seen in the pictures. We started chatting and she said she had done Weight Watchers, and she was playing on three different recreational sports teams! I was even more shocked at that news.

Her playing on three sports teams, in my mind, would be like me deciding tomorrow to try out for a musical. It would be so far outside my comfort zone and would leave me so vulnerable that I honestly would not even think of it.

I asked her why she joined the leagues. She said it went back to the physical education class at our high school. She said that the environment was so supportive and never competitive. It included the non-athletic people as much as the athletes and encouraged participation more than results.

I thought back to our phys. ed. class and I remember playing "Rubber Chicken Basketball"... yes, you read that correctly. In this game, a rubber chicken replaced the ball, and all basketball rules applied, except for dribbling. Shooting and passing were difficult, as was trying not to laugh as someone tried to lob a long pass to a player running up the court. There would be just a rubber chicken flapping in the air, falling way too short of the intended player. This activity promoted teamwork, exercise, and basic movement more than skill. The score was never recorded, and by the end of the game, our faces all hurt from smiling and laughing. That was a well-designed physical education class that had a long-term impact.

My friend, the one-time elite athlete, is now only watching his sport on the television while my other non-athletic friend is playing recreational sport three days a week. Keep these stories in mind when you are gearing up your child for their next sports game or competition. It isn't just okay to have fun, it is the reason they got involved in the first place and it is what will make it a lifelong behaviour.

References

1. Bandura, A. (1977). *Social Learning Theory*. New York: General Learning Press.

2. Fredricks, J & JS Eccles. (2004). Parental Influences on Youth Involvement in Sports. In MR Weiss (Ed.), *Developmental Sport and Exercise Psychology: A Lifespan Perspective* (pp. 145–64). Morgantown, WV: Fitness Information Technology.

Chapter 4

Making Healthy Choices *Easy* Choices

"...life is going to end sooner or later. It's a simple idea, but it's something that always gives me guidance and leads me in the right direction in any moment of confusion or decision. Once you accept that this life will end it then becomes all about experiences.... It does become a little easier to go with the flow and try new things when you accept that our time here is limited." — Richard Bodnuruk

Being faced with death gives us a completely different perspective on life. Few understand this better than Richard Bodnuruk. Serving in the military at a young age, he grew beyond his years, learning exactly what matters to him in life. His body was what would bring him to the highest mountains and carry him toward his goals, whether it was to run an ultra-marathon, travel to 18 more countries, or enjoy time with friends and family. Rich broke free from the cycle of obesity that runs in his family. He took control because he knows he needs a healthy body in order to live the most of every day. He now spends his days motivating others to do the same. To conclude this chapter, we will take a look at many of the factors in our environment that influence our ability to make the healthy choices the easy choices in our lives, and provide ideas for how you can take control of your environment to live life to the fullest every day.

Richard's Story

What is my motivation for living well?

Before I talk about my own story in a little more detail, I'd like to tell you about my background to help you better understand my point of view. I am a 24-year-old co-owner of CrossFit Lazarus, a physical training facility in Edmonton, Alberta, that my partner and I opened with no previous business school training or experience. So far I have racked up a year and a half at the University of Alberta, four years working more than ten jobs in various fields, five and a half years in the army reserve, and a tour of duty to Afghanistan with Task Force 3-09 as a member of the Kandahar Provincial Reconstruction Team (KPRT). A Canadian by birth, I spent five years of my childhood in Bangladesh; my travel résumé includes 18 countries and over half of them I visited on my own.

My story is one that I'm sure is fairly common. As a teenager I had no clue about how to look after my body and I found myself worrying about the bulge sticking out of the middle of my shirt and my cheeks. It wasn't a blinding thought, but it was constant. I hadn't been taught about health and fitness, so I did what all un-knowledgeable people do—I made assumptions. I assumed that some people are just born different and that's just the way it is. I figured that I was a bit bigger, and that some people were bigger than me, some smaller. I didn't have a clue what that meant, what caused the difference, what were better options, or what would produce more desirable outcomes.

I am lucky, however, because I made an important discovery during my teen years. My discovery happened following a season of lacrosse in a new division. By the end of the lacrosse season, more than a few people were commenting on my physical appearance. I realized that I had lost body fat and was looking more like the smaller guys than the bigger ones. I concluded that something I did during the games lead to my positive result. The games consisted of me running after or away from people, and so I concluded that running was to thank for the positive results, and so I should run. So I did.

At first, after a couple of laps around the track, I would have to stop. I didn't understand why I couldn't keep going or what it meant or how to fix it. And I didn't worry about it. I just ran. Eventually magic happened. I could run farther without stopping. And more magic happened—I lost more and more weight. The outcome prompted me to gain the knowledge that I was lacking; I learned why things were happening after the fact and "the magic" that I thought was happening was being replaced in my head with scientific fact.

It was also during my teen years that I began to learn about the role that food plays in body composition. After tearing three ligaments in my left knee in a lacrosse game, I found myself home from school for two straight weeks to recover. To make sure I was able to keep up my grades, my science teacher gave me an upcoming assignment early. The teacher told me to track my food intake for a week straight, put my results in a calculator that looked at macro- and micronutrient levels, and hand in the results. This was my first look at nutrition and the real breakdown of food. This process completely opened my eyes to the idea that food is a fuel and that my seemingly unrelated weight loss and fitness results were actually completely dependant on it. Once I combined this nutritional information with the workout knowledge I had gained until that point, I saw my weight go from 200 to 160 lbs over the period of a year and a half and then back up to a very different looking 190 lbs.

My initial inspiration was at the time unknown to me. But as I progressed, my inspiration and motivation evolved, as did my success. As I became more fit I started looking into things that became available thanks to my fitness. Fitness gave me new inspiration to get even more fit and caused me to accomplish more, which allowed me to explore new adventures, such as scuba diving, climbing mountains, and sports.

A couple of years later, I found myself with new motivation as I began getting ready for deployment to Afghanistan with the military. It was obvious from the start of my pre-training what had to happen for me to get ready physically, and it was clear that I wouldn't be as fit as I wanted to be before deployment, despite my best efforts. I decided then to work intelligently in order to accomplish as much as I could. Many of my fellow soldiers were curious about the work I was doing and began to look to me for advice. When the people who will be responsible for dragging you away from danger ask you how to do it most effectively, you learn how to teach! Fast. That was how I found my inspiration to share my training knowledge. At the time, I was simply interested in helping some soldiers get a little bit better at exercising and getting more fit. What I got out of it was the ability to teach. Eventually this process got better and better as I got more used to teaching, and as it became easier I wanted to do it more and more. Success breeds success, which is an idea that provides motivation and inspiration to any aspect of life.

Now it's hard for me to imagine a quality life that doesn't involve training. Preparing for combat has allowed me to develop a body with a lot more potential than before. Now, without the stress of combat, a few things keep me motivated to keep it going. I have found like-minded people who have similar outlooks and goals, and this community has been a huge motivator for me.

My motivation to join the military from the start was simply the adventure and experience, and a fortunate series of events supported this. I was there for the experience, and it was the only goal that I had. This mindset has transferred to my life after Afghanistan. Shortly after I came home, a stint of boredom prompted me to book a flight to Peru leaving ten days later. I lured a friend of mine with the promise of adventure, and a couple days later we were off on our impromptu trip. The result of that trip was more than a high-altitude tan. A day after we descended the ruins of Machu Picchu, we found ourselves at a playground in Cusco doing a workout, and soon a handful of Peruvian children joined us. On the plane ride back to Canada, with the memory of coaching six Peruvian kids in broken Spanish to pump out pushups, the idea for our gym CrossFit Lazarus was born. Soon something we had merely chatted about became an instant reality, and we saw how possible it actually was. In a couple of minutes we had inspired those kids to copy us, had shown them how to do things properly, and then watched as they took off on their own. By the time we had left the park, they were still going, and we were left wondering how much more of an impact we could make. A seemingly carefree trip with a friend would be responsible for changing the parameters of my life and career.

We didn't realize then what we would create in the next couple of months and what the next two years would look like for us. One thing slowly lead to another; conversations turned into reality. A small idea was combined with another one until months and months passed and we began to look at a complex business that was growing and evolving every day. Our gym is more than an idea thrown around in a conversation—now it's a physical place. The cliché you would expect to hear from a gym owner is of empowerment and life-changing experiences, which seems mildly impressive on paper. It is, however, incredible when you see it happen before your eyes. We see changes daily: We see people succeed and fail; people battle themselves, their emotions, self-worth issues, their wants, and their needs. We expected people to lose weight and get stronger with CrossFit—that's a simple equation. We didn't expect people to tell us that because of our gym, Edmonton began to feel like home for them, that the community we created had been essential in getting them through the months of a terminally sick parent, or that our gym was the first thing to excite their spouse after ten years of trying new hobbies and interests and that it has strengthened their relationship. I didn't expect my own mom, who had been experiencing age-related injuries and falls, to start coming three times a week, lose 30 lbs, and be able to lift 125 lbs.

This idea of adventures producing unforeseen positive results is a consistent in my life and is something I believe lends itself to a fulfilled and happy life. I like to give myself new "good stress" by constantly trying new challenges or setting somewhat unrealistic goals to keep me going. My most recent goal was to attempt to run a 125K ultra-marathon for the first time without ever competing in anything over 10K. The outcome of the race was ultimately a failure; with finishing as my goal I fell short by timing out around the 67 km mark. The risk of impending failure is a great motivator, and although 67 km is not 125km, it was significantly farther than I had ever gone before. Both in my travels and in my coaching, I always try to explore new territory.

So here are some of the lessons that have helped me shape my life and have contributed to my current situation:

- Start small. Whatever goal it is you are trying to achieve, if it has any value, likely it will be an overwhelming or daunting task. When you are getting started, the most important thing is to just show up and be open to new ideas. As you spend time working towards your small goals, you will inevitably achieve at least a small measure of success. Success breeds success, and as time goes on, expectations and goals can evolve to match your output.

- Surround yourself with a good group of people. This might be the most important point related to achieving success in any form. If you are surrounded by smart, motivated, and inspired people, they will push you to rise to the occasion and get better. Objectively look at the people in your life and cut back on the time you spend with those who are not bringing you up. At a minimum, identify people are who are negative and uncommitted, so that the next time they discredit the work you are doing, offer you junk food despite knowing your weight loss goal, or bring drama into your personal life when you are trying to get it in order, you will at least know they are trying to derail you and you can treat the situation as such.

- Take strength in role models. If someone inspires you, use it as motivation for your own story. It can be anyone, from movie

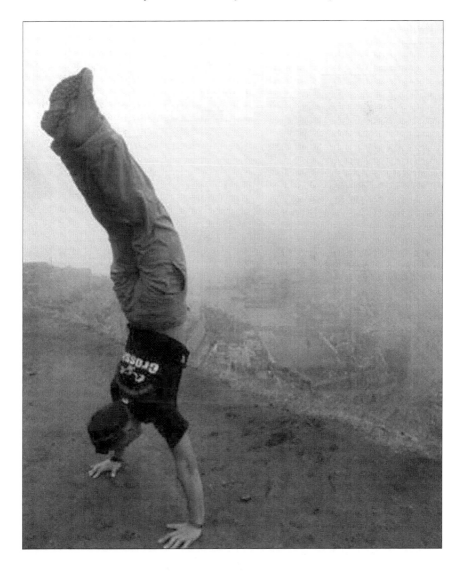

stars and athletes to mentors in your field or friends who are one step ahead of where you are right now. Either way, use someone else's example as proof that it is at very least possible.

- Travel as much as you can in as many ways as you can. Inspiration is out there; you just have to find it.

- Accept that you won't be able to plan for everything. Be willing to take the risk. Thinking things out is important, but so is action. Take the plunge.

It takes time to not suck at things. Anytime you feel like an idiot when you try something new, it's an investment. It is hard to remain inexperienced when you keep doing something. Look on the bright side. If you start today instead of tomorrow, you'll reach your goal one day sooner.

Changing the Cycle of Obesity: What You Need to Know

Richard discusses his early struggles with body weight and self-image as a teenager; these struggles are becoming increasingly common worldwide among both children and teens. We continue to see an increased number of overweight and obese people across all age groups, particularly here in North America. What we found so inspirational about Richard's story is his ability to use his personal motivation to take control of the factors in his life that dictate his health and well-being. Recognizing the factors within our environment that act as barriers to wellness is an important step in *removing* or *reducing* these barriers to our long-term health. This section will further discuss this topic, provide you with examples of common barriers, and make suggestions for reducing sedentary behaviours and improving the quality of your food choices.

"Obesogenic" Environment

If weight loss were simple, over 60 percent of the North American population wouldn't be overweight or obese.[1-3] The reality is that the current "obesity epidemic" is anything but simple. It is often said that the reason our society struggles with weight is because we are "eating more and moving less," and all that needs to be done to solve the epidemic is to eat less and move more. Although intake and activity certainly are contributing factors, it is not easy to change these behaviours because our intake and physical activity each depend on many factors themselves. With respect to "eating more," we could look at the total number of calories eaten per day, the frequency or pattern of eating, the composition of the food eaten, the amount of processing our food has undergone, additives found in our foods and beverages, the availability of food, social aspects and influences of eating, and so on. For "moving less" we need to consider the total number of minutes of activity per day, the intensity of activity, the type of activity, the long-term frequency or variety of activities performed, and so on. You can see that these two "simple" determinants of body weight in themselves have a lot more to them than you might initially consider.

In addition to diet and exercise, there are many other factors that contribute to body weight that have nothing directly to do with eating or moving. A non-exhaustive list includes genetic predisposition; smoking and alcohol consumption habits; stress level (and how well we cope with stress: see Chapter 10); sleep (see Chapter 10); social supports; your profession; and environmental factors, such as where you live, where you work, your daily commute, food availability, local programs and policy, and your city's infrastructure. Many health professionals believe that it is this overall picture that has changed more significantly than how *much* we eat or move. Many feel that our environment promotes obesity and that we live in a so-called "obesogenic environment." In one excellent resource, Dr. Rebecca Lee, professor in the department of health and human performance at the University of Houston, writes extensively about this very subject in her book *Reversing the Obesogenic Environment*.[4] For example, one chapter examines the various environmental factors that influence our decisions to take part in physical activity: such factors include accessibility, proximity, safety, features, amenities, quality and condition of facilities, walking paths, bike trails, and other resources within a community intended for promoting physical activity.

The Role of Exercise in Weight Management

I have to start this section off with a very important statement: You can out eat any exercise plan. I first heard this statement from one of my undergraduate professors, Dr. Angie Thompson, and I was devastated. I grew up with the very convenient notion that I could eat anything that I wanted to because I was active. As Dr. Thompson pointed out in that lecture, it is much easier and can be more enjoyable to sit down and consume calories than it is to expend them. Throw in the fact that our society focuses celebrations, life events, family time, social time, and business meetings all around food, and it just adds to the problem. (To be fair, it is extremely difficult to host a budget meeting soccer game, so serving food does make more sense.) For this reason, engaging in physical activity during your recreation time and wherever it can fit into your life is extremely important.

The Role of Exercise in Body Composition

As explained above, being overweight and obese has become an epidemic. Carrying around excess fat can be a massive burden on your body and is associated with the development of many chronic diseases, such as hypertension, heart disease, diabetes, cancer, and sleep apnea, many of which can be deadly. This epidemic stresses our health care system and costs taxpayers billions of dollars. (The Public Health Agency of Canada has stated that the economic costs of obesity are on the rise, at an estimated $4.6 billion in 2008 and close to $7 billion in indirect costs associated with treatment of chronic diseases linked to obesity.[1]) On a personal level, obesity limits what activities people can enjoy, affects movement, and restricts what people can do with their lives.

Exercise can help with weight loss, but more importantly and more dramatically, it can contribute to the health of body. Exercise can improve or help to maintain lean body mass (muscle), improve insulin sensitivity, favourably change metabolic rate, improve mood, and reduce many of the obesity-related comorbidities listed above. See page 67 for a chart showing the different heart rate zones for different training goals (i.e., fat burning versus endurance training).

Following exercise, energy expenditure remains elevated above pre-exercise levels because you are burning even more calories at rest. This depends of course on the type and intensity of the exercise, slightly less on the duration.

A great example of the power of exercise occurs in diabetics. Regular aerobic exercise can lower your blood sugar level without medication and can help burn excess calories and fat to manage weight. Exercise decreases insulin resistance *even in the absence of weight loss*. Exercise also increases the body's energy level, lowers tension, and improves the ability to handle stress. Many people with type 2 diabetes can discontinue medication altogether and manage the disease based on lifestyle changes alone (exercise and proper nutrition).[5]

I use diabetes and obesity as examples of the power of exercise. If you are not diabetic or obese, exercise is still a very powerful behaviour. Exercise is the "output" for energy balance, and since we are consuming calories on a daily basis, exercise is important for weight management and weight loss.

When you exercise regularly your body will function better, right down to the cellular level. As expressed in the diabetes example, exercise can decrease insulin resistance, literally changing your body's ability to use insulin, a hormone needed for the body to properly use sugars as a source of energy. Exercise can lower the amount of cortisol (the stress hormone) in our bodies, which can reduce wear and tear on almost all of our body's systems and even make our skin look younger. I could go on and on about the benefits of exercise, but the truth of the matter is that if you want your body to work properly, you need to move it.

The current physical activity guidelines in both Canada and the US recommend *at least* 150 minutes of moderate physical activity a week. Note that this guideline serves as a minimum. For individuals who would like to see weight loss and increased health benefits from physical activity, the American College of Sports Medicine recommends individuals slowly work up to 200 to 300 minutes (3.3 to 5 hours) of moderate activity per week.[6] The majority of this activity should be aerobic, keeping an elevated heart rate for a period of time, such as brisk walking, jogging, or riding a bike.

IMPORTANT: Proper weight loss takes time and is a complete lifestyle change, something you will need to maintain for the rest of your life. People do not typically gain weight over a short period of time, so you cannot expect to lose it in a short period of time with any chance at maintaining the change. A combination approach of both exercise and nutrition is ideal with high motivation and social support. Weight loss is not easy and in our current society requires a lot of will power and planning ahead.

References

1. Obesity in Canada. (2011). A joint report from the Public Health Agency of Canada and the Canadian Institute for Health Information. Available online at: www.phac-aspc.gc.ca/hp-ps/hl-mvs/oic-oac/assets/pdf/oic-oac-eng.pdf.

2. Centers for Disease Control and Prevention. (January 2012). Prevalence of Obesity in the United States, 2009-2010 (Data from the NHANES). Available online at: www.cdc.gov/nchs/data/databriefs/db82.pdf.

3. Ogden, CL & MD Carroll. (2010). Prevalence of Overweight, Obesity, and

Extreme Obesity Among Adults: United States, Trends 1960–1962 Through 2007–2008. Centers for Disease Control and Prevention. Available online at: www.cdc.gov/nchs/fastats/overwt.htm.

4. Lee, R, K McAlexander, & J Banda. (2011). _Reversing the Obesogenic Environment._ Champaign, IL: Human Kinetics.

5. Durstine, JL, G Moore, P Painter, & S Roberts. (2009). _ACSM's Exercise Management for Persons with Chronic Diseases and Disabilities._ (3d Ed.) Champaign, IL: Human Kinetics.

6. Donnelly, JE et al. (2009). Appropriate physical activity intervention strategies for weight loss and prevention of weight regain for adults. _Medicine & Science in Sport & Exercise_ 41(2). pp 459-71.

Chapter 5

Charting Your Course: Getting Back to Basics

"I was seventy-five pounds overweight, was struggling with acid reflux, had a persistent cough, and required increasing amounts of pain medication. For the first time in my life, I made a New Year's resolution to get fit and lose weight. This is a lifestyle change." — Judy Yawney

As a home economist and volunteer coordinator for Edmonton's Food Bank, Judy Yawney sees the difficulties of food insecurity and lack of skills for food preparation on a daily basis. Despite her healthy upbringing, Judy struggled with her own weight and health issues for years following an injury that resulted from a motor vehicle incident while she was cycling. This all changed for her when she made a New Year's resolution to radically transform her own diet and lifestyle for the long term. She has made a brave and successful return to commuting by bicycle and supports initiatives throughout the country that focus on healthy lifestyle practices. Following Judy's story we will discuss aspects of eating and physical activity that Judy uses to promote her long-term health, including meal planning basics and a variety of ways to track your activity in order to continuously challenge your body.

Judy's Story: A New Year's Resolution to Last a Lifetime

My name is Judy Yawney and I am the Volunteer Coordinator at Edmonton's Food Bank. I graduated from the University of Alberta with a BSc in Home Economics in 1986. As I write this, I think of the interesting twists and turns and even detours my life has taken over the last 50 plus years.

Having grown up in Rossland, British Columbia, I had a relatively active lifestyle of swimming, cycling, and hiking in the summer and, of course, downhill skiing at Red Mountain in the winter. In 1981, all that changed for me.

I was in motor vehicle accident while cycling and suffered massive pelvic and spinal injuries. After nine weeks in the hospital and two years of physiotherapy, my active lifestyle was no longer very active. With each passing year, it became more difficult to be active and maintain my health. I dreaded shopping for clothes, as nothing ever fit me! There was also a cloud of a family history of diabetes hanging over my head. Plus the driver who changed my life was also diabetic! (The driver had cataracts and diabetic retinopathy.)

On New Year's Day 2007, I came to understand that I had to make some drastic changes in my lifestyle. I was 75 lbs overweight, was struggling with acid reflux, had a persistent cough, and required increasing amounts of pain medication. With a family history of both type 1 and 2 diabetes, the change became even more critical. As well, my nephew, who was in his 30s had recently been diagnosed with type 1 diabetes.

What changed that day in 2007?

For the first time in my life, I made a New Year's resolution to get fit and lose weight. Since then, I have participated in the Running Room's Resolution Run/Walk , which helps me to stay focused on this promise to myself.

Most importantly, I am eating healthy! I always have lots of fresh fruit and vegetables in my fridge, and pack a sensible lunch for work each day. I also support local food producers through farmers' markets. I have to admit, however, that I sometimes have trouble drinking enough water, as I'm on my feet at work for hours at a time!

Portion control and meal planning have been essential. On weekends, I prepare meals that I am able to reheat for dinners or take as leftovers. I shop for groceries only once each week and always with a list that I stick to. When I started shopping once a week, I found I had more disposable income as well! I also make it a rule not to eat within the last three hours before going to bed.

Exercise has become part of my daily routine. I wear my pedometer to track how many steps I take, with an average of between 15,000 to 22,000 steps per day.

Although I had always enjoyed cycling, I was terrified to return to it after my accident. With some help and encouragement from friends, I started biking again. Initially, I would only cycle on trails. I am gradually gaining my confidence and becoming a bit more adventurous after participating in the MS Bike Tour (190K) the last few summers (and I'm hoping to register for next year). I have also explored some of the Kettle Valley Railway in southern BC (and even had a close encounter with a bear).

In addition, I've also started cycling to work— seven kilometres each way. I even cycle to work during the winter, as I am fortunate to be able to use the incredible trail system here in Edmonton. This last summer, I even took a women's mountain bike clinic in Fernie, BC. And yes, I have returned to downhill skiing, gradually making my way back to the black diamond runs! I have also participated in the Rossland tradition of hiking Mount Roberts in the Rossland Range for Canada Day (a 7.5K hike with a change in elevation of 860 metres).

Since January 2007, I have lost 65 lbs and now require minimal pain medication. In fact, I recently had to replace all my pain medication, as they had all expired. With a healthy diet, following *Canada's Food Guide*, I find I have control of my acid reflux without having to take medication, since it was acidic foods and fats that were the culprits for me. My persistent cough has disappeared.

As a home economist, I am alarmed by the number of people today who are unable to make simple meals and are reliant on convenience foods. Add to that the increasing rate of type 2 diabetes and inactivity, and the importance of a healthy lifestyle becomes all the more evident, which will impact our health care system. Some local initiatives I support include community gardens and Plant a Row, Grow a Row, which encourages individuals to plant an extra row of produce to support their local food banks. (For more information on this program, please contact your local food bank.)

I've realized that eating healthy and daily exercise is a lifestyle change, which will be with me for life!

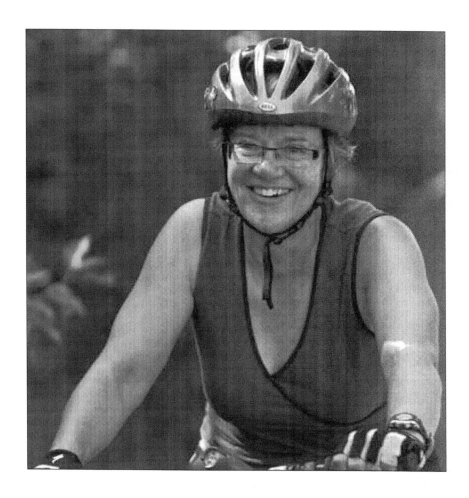

Back to Basics: Meal Planning 101

"He who fails to plan is planning to fail" — Winston Churchill

I completely agree with Judy's statement that the lack of meal planning and cooking skills found in many people is alarming. Based on my experience, many of us use lack of time as an excuse to reach for convenience foods throughout the day. Realistically though, a few simple planning tools will help get you on the right track. The first step is to plan your meals. Taking just 15 minutes once a week before grocery shopping to decide what you want to eat for each meal in the upcoming week will save you time and money (and the urge to order take-out). Planning will also help you to create a grocery list to ensure that you've got all the required ingredients and avoid extra trips to the store throughout the week that waste time and gas money. You'll also save money by purchasing ingredients to make recipes from scratch rather than relying on food that is already prepared. You pay a premium for pre-prepared items or sauces, and these often contain high amount of salt, sugar, or fat (or all three). Finally, planning in advance helps to minimize waste, which keeps even more of your hard-earned money in your pocket.

When meal planning, keep a few things in mind:

- Write down what you'd like to eat for each meal throughout the week. (If you're just starting out, you could try just doing this for the supper meals.) Then prepare your grocery list by going through the meals and writing down the items you need to purchase in order to make each meal. See the example below.

- Incorporate three or four food groups to make balanced meals that provide a wide array of nutrients. Each food group contains vitamins and minerals that are in lesser quantities or may be absent from another food group, so incorporating more food groups brings a well-rounded plate of nutrients to your body. For example, grain products are typically high in B-vitamins; meat and alternatives (such as beans, lentils, and tofu) are sources of iron and zinc; milk and milk alternatives (such as fortified soy or almond beverages) contain much more calcium per serving than other food groups; and vegetables and fruit contain a wide array of antioxidant vitamins.

- For an extra nutritional boost, plan to include at least two food groups into each snack that you might consume during the day. Good choices would be veggie sticks or whole wheat pitas and hummus, or yogurt with fruit.

- Use recipes while meal planning, especially if you're trying something new. This will ensure that you have all necessary ingredients on hand.

- Another time-saving tool for making healthy food choices is to prepare extra servings of your dinner each night to use as a quick and healthy leftover lunch for the following day.

- Involve the whole family! Including your partner, roommate, or children allows the whole household to be engaged in planning for healthy eating. This sets a great example for kids and teaches the importance of including variety in our diet. They also might want to help participate in the preparation or cooking process. For example, allowing children to wash fruit and vegetables or scrub potatoes, and teaching teens to chop and dice foods, will prepare the next generation with skills for lifelong healthy eating.

Taking the time to plan meals will add up to major time and cost savings throughout the week.

If you're struggling with the same boring rotation of meals, try something new! Most of us only have a rotation of a few meals that we make regularly. Spice things up by adding some variety. Ask friends and family for their favourite recipes or borrow a cookbook for inspiration. Starting an email recipe exchange with friends, family, or co-workers can also be a fun way to gather new ideas (see the template below). Another way to get ideas is to join (or start) a community cooking club. These clubs bring groups of individuals together from a community. Each person brings in his or her favourite recipe at the beginning of the season, and the group takes turns each week cooking each recipe as a group. At the end of each class, you'll have learned and sampled another member's recipe. It's a great social activity and a fun way to try new recipes and gain new culinary skills!

Meal Planning Example

Sunday
Breakfast: scrambled eggs, toast, and yogurt parfait
* *Groceries needed: eggs, bread, yogurt, frozen berries, granola*
Lunch: tuna sandwich, veggies and dip, fruit, glass of milk
* *Groceries needed: bread, canned light tuna, dressing/dip, carrots, cucumber, celery, grapes, milk*
Supper: chicken stir-fry
* *Groceries needed: chicken breasts, rice, broccoli, carrots, water chestnuts, bell peppers, teriyaki sauce*

Repeat for each day. For snacks, think about what you'd like to include throughout the week and write these down at the end.

Here is an example of a popular **email recipe exchange template** (as the first to send this, have a friend start the chain with you by placing your friend's email address in position 1 and your email address in position 2; then send BCC or blind copy to 20 friends, colleagues, or family members):

Please join in on a collective and delicious adventure: You are invited to participate in a recipe exchange. I hope you will participate!

Please send a recipe to the person whose email address is in position 1 below (even if you don't know him/her); it should be something quick, easy, and without hard-to-find ingredients. This could be one you've memorized and can type right now. Don't agonize over it; it is one you make when you are short on time (or something extra tasty that you always get compliments on!).

After you've sent your recipe to the email address listed in position 1 below, and only to that person, copy this letter into a new email and move my email address to position 1 and put your email address in position 2. Only our two email addresses should show when you send your email.

Send to 20 friends BCC (blind copy) who you think would like to participate. If you're unable to do this within one week, let me know so it will be fair to those participating. It's fun to see where they come from and the variety of recipes you'll receive! Seldom does anyone drop out because we all need new ideas. The turnaround is fast, as there are only two names on the list and you only have to do it once.

Position 1: example@gmail.com
Position 2: example@hotmail.com

Tracking the Way You Move

In Judy's story she talks about the number of steps she was tracking with her pedometer, which is a small device that can be placed on your hip to track how many steps you take each day. Having some sort of objective way to measure your activity level can be motivational, and for the "data junkies" of the world it offers concrete objective information on your exercise.

Burke et al. (2011) reported that self-reporting physical activity at least once a week was associated with performing more exercise.[1]

They also suggest that people should record time, intensity, and frequency for exercise. This review concludes that self-monitoring exercise, diet, and weight are effective ways to increase exercise, healthy eating, and weight loss.

Pedometers

Keeping track of your exercise gives you a great indicator of where you are now, allows you to make a specific goal (see Chapter 12), and to progress to your goal. For example, for health benefits it is suggested you take at least 10,000 steps each day. If you are using a pedometer, you might notice you are only taking 6,000 steps a day (most people are surprised how few steps they take daily). Start recording how many steps you are doing daily (daily step counting sheet available at *www.inspiremewell.com*). You can begin to do activities to increase your steps. The pedometer is a tool that provides you with real-time honest feedback about your activity, and can serve as an excellent motivational tool to increase your activity level.

I have a 72-year-old client who wears a pedometer everyday. If, at dinner, she notices she does not have enough steps, she will go for a walk around her block or actually do laps inside the house. She has also adopted some habits to increase her steps. For example, she will park farther away from the store to have a longer walk. She also takes the stairs whenever she can.

Journaling

If you have ever watched the show *House* you will know the main character, Dr. House, often says "everybody lies." This is very true with exercise. It is a well-known fact that when researchers ask people how much exercise they are doing, most people overestimate their activity and the intensity at which it is performed. Keep track of your exercise by writing it down either in a journal, your agenda, or one of the many online resources, such as *fitday.com*, to track, share, and compare your progress

Apps

There are now countless apps available for your smart phone or tablet that allow you to keep track of activity. Many use GPS and can give you a very precise way to measure distance, time, speed, and calories burned if you go for a walk, run, or bike ride. For many people this is a great way to keep track of their activity, as they are never more than an arm's length away from their phones.

Gadgets

There are numerous gadgets out there that track the very details of your activity. These high-tech toys can be watches (Garmin), or devices placed in or on your shoes (Nike+, Adidas miCoach), around your waist, or taped to your thigh (research-grade accelerometers). Many of these can be connected to a smart phone or to your computer. Using these devices, you can acquire information about pretty much anything you need to know for your training… and then some.

For many of these gadgets, there are also online communities set up where you can upload and share your data. These communities act as a virtual support system where you can share, compare, and inspire others. When you know you are being measured or know you have someone to be accountable to, you may be more apt to push yourself further.

Heart Rate

The proper intensity of exercise is extremely important to achieve maximum health and training benefits. Many gadgets have the technology to track intensity, but if you do not have these gadgets or are not tech savvy, there are other ways to monitor how you are doing. Taking it from high-tech to basic, your heart rate is the best way to keep track of your intensity. You can track your heart by using a heart rate monitor (around your torso), built-in monitors on aerobic machines, or by taking your pulse. You must maintain a heart rate in the Target Heart Rate Zone (THRZ) for the allotted time in order to gain the most benefit from your exercise. Your target heart rate zone will depend on your goals.

A simple way to calculate an your heart rate max is:
220 minus (-) your age = your heart rate maximum

Here is an example for a 30-year-old:
220 - 30(years) = maximum heart rate is 190 beats per minute (bpm)

Now that you have your maximum heart rate (Max HR %), you can train at different levels of that max based on your goals.

Exercise Level	Benefits	Intensity (Max HR %)
Light exercise	Healthy heart maintenance	50%-60%
Weight loss	Burning fat	60%-70%
Aerobic	Endurance	70%-80%
Conditioning	Muscle building	80%-90%
Athlete	Athletic training	90% and above

Choose your intensity and then calculate your target heart rate range. Using the same example of a 30-year-old looking to work in the *aerobic* target heart rate zone:

190bpm x 70% = 133bpm
190bpm x 80% = 152bpm
Target heart rate range = 133bpm–152bpm

How to take your own pulse:
- On your wrist: With palm up, place your finger on the thumb

side of your wrist, about one inch below the wrist joint.

- On your neck: The main artery to the head runs next to the windpipe, below the ear. Using one of these locations, count the number of beats in ten seconds then multiply that number by six. This will give you your bpms for all your intensity calculations if you do not have access to a heart rate monitor.

If you find it difficult taking your own pulse, you can use the Borg rate of perceived exertion (RPE) scale. This is a scale from 6 to 20. Six is equivalent to just sitting and relaxing, while 20 is running from a bear and turning blue (maximal effort). As you get used to the scale, the numbers will be approximately equivalent to your heartbeat. Six will correspond to about 60 beats per minute, 7 to about 70 beats per minute, and so on. This is a crude estimate, but it will allow you to approximate your effort and to see improvements as your fitness improves.

6	No exertion (sitting/relaxing)
7	Extremely light
8	
9	Very light
10	
11	Light
12	
13	Somewhat Hard
14	
15	Hard
16	
17	Very Hard
18	
19	Extremely Hard
20	Maximal Exertion

Whichever way works best for you, be sure to track your activity and your progress as you move towards your goal. Share your progress with others if you need a little push. You can also use the systems, technologies, and concepts mentioned above to create a detailed plan for physical activity (see Chapter 12).

References

1. Burke, LE et al. Using mHealth Technology to Enhance Self-Monitoring for Weight Loss: A Randomized Trial. *Am J Prev Med*. 2012 Jul; 43(1): 20-26.

Chapter 6

Healthy Healing: Overcoming Trauma and Taking Control

"For a long time I used food to hide myself from the past of being abused. I thought that eating and being bigger would keep men away from me and from abusing me."
— Glori Meldrum

Glori Meldrum's story is both tragic and heroic; it is also more common than we would like to think. Through difficult situations, it becomes increasingly important to take care of your health both physically and psychologically. Both of these components are important, and we often forget how interconnected they are. Many people are self-medicating, using food as an antidepressant and anti-anxiety tool, and are under-using exercise. This not only negatively affects our physical health, but also our self-esteem and energy levels, and it tends to become a downward spiral leading to more food and less activity. Eating well and exercising are not the only things you can do to get through a difficult situation or trauma. They can also be something to use to cope with future hardships by providing both physical and mental strength, resilience, and perseverance.

Glori's Story

For my children, for my husband, for the eight-year-old me.

I was born in 1973 and grew up on both coasts before I finally made my home in Edmonton, Alberta. I was born to run. As far back as I can remember, I was always pushing myself to achieve—

not just on the race track, but also in my personal life, my career, and my charitable service. The trophies I've claimed thus far include my wonderful husband Gary, my three children, my several businesses (including g[squared] and Trafik Interactive), and the personal fulfillment that's come from my work in Africa and with Little Warriors. Though my race is far from over, I wake up each day knowing I have already won.

Although I am thankful every day for all the wonderful people and treasures in my life; it is truly a contrast to the nightmare of my childhood. On December 31, 1981, when I was eight years old, a family member sexually abused me for the first time. This abuse continued for the next couple of years. When I finally told my mother what had happened, she took me to social services, but when they interviewed my abuser, he denied it and they took him at his word. No charges were laid against him and my accusation tore my family apart. It would take 25 years before my abuser saw a courtroom, but—in my case—justice has still yet to be served due to an absurd legal technicality.

Denied closure by our legal system, I realized that it was up to me to tend to my own psychological wounds. It was time for me to learn how to love myself. Finding the strength I needed to do this through my exploration of spirituality and yoga, I discovered my true purpose in life: to live a life of service by helping and healing others and doing everything I can to eradicate the scourge of child sexual abuse.

It's one thing to discover your life's purpose; it's another to do something about it. In my case, I formed Little Warriors in 2007. It's a charity dedicated to preventing child sexual abuse through awareness and the promotion of adult education.

While my life is full of my passions, it is also very busy. When asked about my wellness, I thought of a lesson I learned recently. For many years I ran on the treadmill of life at full speed. I never stopped; I just kept running. I would run so fast I would trigger my anxiety and I would end up very sick. Once I had enough energy to function I would run again and fast. I never took breaks or enjoyed much of anything. I was very sick in many ways. In the last few months, I have started to get very run down. I have felt overwhelmed about raising money for Little Warriors and finding money to build the Be Brave Ranch, a place for child and adult survivors of child sexual abuse. Being in this place of being overwhelmed, I triggered my anxiety in a bad way. However, recently I did something I have never done when I started to fall off the treadmill: I hit the stop button and got off. I took a few days off and cared for myself.

I know you're asking: "You mean we can actually get off the treadmill?" Yes, we can. We just have to hit the stop button and get off. I did. I am the type of person who gives everything they have when they take on something, even if they end up really sick. So this time I got off the treadmill and made a commitment not to take everything on myself. Little Warriors is not mine, it is OURS. Little Warriors belongs to Canadians, and if we want to build the Be Brave Ranch and we want Little Warriors to do great things, then we all have to support it in whatever way we can. We cannot just talk about it. My dream is to build the Be Brave Ranch, but I cannot do it alone. I am very proud of the lesson of stepping off the treadmill. I have also learned that I am only one person and I need help. I am going to take better care of myself.

Without my health there would be no me: no companies, no mother for my children, and no passions. Self-care is so important. For a long time I used food to hide myself from the past of being abused. I thought that eating and being bigger would keep men away from me and from abusing me. Over the past couple of years, I went from being a size 14 to a size 4 and I feel great. I started doing Moksha Yoga several times a week, although keeping up with three children is a workout of its own. I want to be around for my children, and my grandchildren someday, and of course my husband. I have to say, having a supportive husband helps so much.

He motivates the whole family to make healthy choices.

I was able to find the tools I needed to survive my own personal nightmare. Sadly, many other survivors of child sexual abuse haven't yet found these tools. My dream is to build the Little Warriors Be Brave Ranch, a spiritual oasis where a neglected survivor can be given the tools they need to heal their body, heart, spirit, and mind.

For more information on Little Warriors and Glori Meldrum, please visit *www.littlewarriors.ca.*

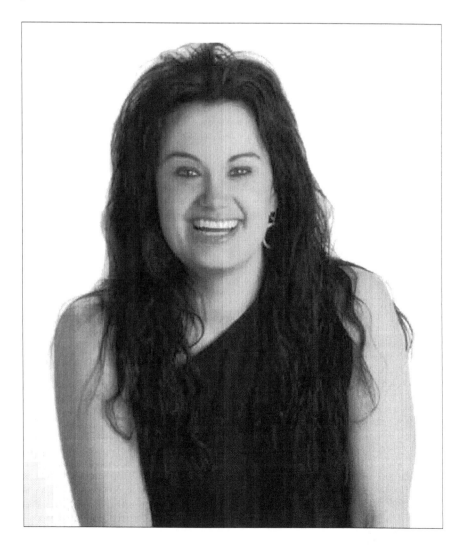

Yoga: Exploring the Edge

Glori discusses using yoga as part of her process, which made me curious to explore yoga as a method of recovery. Anyone who has ever done yoga can confidently say "it makes me feel better." Perhaps you cannot put your finger on the exact reason why. I was the same way. I absolutely love my morning yoga class—even if there are times when I have no idea how I am going to get out of some of those positions. I even kept my affection for yoga after I face-planted in the sand while attempting an arm balance while I was in Mexico. My dignity was gone, but my love for yoga remained. Yoga has been an Eastern tradition for thousands of years and is well-known to improve health. Being a researcher, however, that is not enough for me. Why is it effective? Why does it make us feel better?

I started to search the literature and was shocked and impressed on how many studies have been done to investigate the benefits of yoga. It has been credited for increasing energy, aiding in weight loss, increasing biomarkers in the immune system, and increasing our ability to tolerate pain. I am really not too sure these studies were needed though: If you have ever seen the yogis sit on snow with bare skin for hours, you know there is a mind-body connection that is beyond comprehension.

There are even studies examining the benefits of yoga in specific populations. For example, my research experience with yoga included being involved in a study with Iyengar yoga and breast cancer survivors.[1] This study found that the women who participated in the yoga program had significant improvements in quality of life, had increased happiness, and had decreased levels of fatigue This may not be surprising to most, but take a minute to think about how valuable this is. Quality of life encompasses both physical and mental well-being and is the most desired outcome for most pharmaceutical trials. If a drug company could develop a drug to improve the quality of life of a certain disease population, they would be thrilled and every physician would prescribe it. Yoga is able to do this, without drugs, and the list of side effects are things such as better range of motion, greater flexibility, aid in weight maintenance, and the list goes on.

Yoga has demonstrated some of the same benefits as other forms of exercise; however, it comes with an added benefit, especially to the psyche, because of the mind-body connection emphasized in yogic practice. In Western society we often treat the mind and the body ailments separately despite their being so intertwined. How can we ever isolate one from the other? This becomes increasingly evident in trauma survivors.

The effects of yoga have also been studied in people with post-traumatic stress disorder (PTSD). For example, a three-year National Institute of Health (NIH)-funded study examined the effect of yoga on treatment-resistant PTSD and demonstrated the possibility for yoga to have a tremendous impact on these people. Trauma-informed gentle yoga can lead to a significant reduction in symptoms of PTSD, including a reduction of intrusive thoughts, and less dissociation from the body. After the study, which lasted ten weeks, several women no longer had the diagnosis criteria for PTSD.[2]

Why does yoga have such an impact? Most experts and trauma survivors agree, trauma can continue to live in the body and can appear as headaches, twitches, muscle tension, inflammatory responses, and panic attacks, among many other physical symptoms. These "issues in our tissues," as dubbed by Linda Sparrowe, former managing editor of *Yoga Journal* and yoga teacher, can dramatically affect every aspect of trauma survivors' lives. The suggestion has been made that a better approach to therapy could be psychotherapy (traditional talk therapy) combined with a yoga practice. This combination approach allows for healing of both the mind and the body.

When I asked Sparrowe about yoga and trauma, she explained how victims can explore their bodies on their yoga mats in a safe environment. In many trauma cases, the survivors of sexual assault, cancer, or even war experience a body-mind disconnect or are "locked out" of their bodies. On your mat you can explore your edge, hold your edge for a few seconds, and notice but not react to the discomfort.

In one morning class, my teacher said something that opened my eyes to the parallel of life and yoga. The word *yoga* means union. The practice of yoga encourages you to witness your thoughts and your bodily sensations but not react to them. When we were in a particularly difficult position, my instructor said:

Notice what your body is feeling, notice where your mind wants to go. In yoga, like life, you find yourself in positions you do not want to be in—you witness them but never get too involved. Breathe through it, and you will be surprised to find your strength.

— Jessica Ferguson, Lotus Soul Gym, Edmonton, Alberta

Yoga is not a pill you can take each morning; you have to *learn* how to control your bodily reflexes. Mindfulness and mediation (the central components of yoga), learning to observe the internal ebb and flow of your body, and staying in the moment are key to the healing of PTSD or anxiety. Keep in mind, with either of these conditions, meditation can be difficult and can take some time to learn. Yoga Nidra (guided meditation) may be a great place to start, as the instructor guides you through the process and encourages the quieting of the roaming mind. Keep with it. Yoga has been shown to rewire the brain and actually change the neural pathways. Variations of Yoga Nidra have been used to treat depression, anxiety, addiction, and chronic diseases and to help with childbirth. Although this section concentrates on yoga and trauma, it is important to note the extensive benefits of yoga for anyone.

"Why do you stay in prison when the door is so wide open?"
— Rumi

If you do not currently participate in a yoga practice, I strongly encourage you try it. Even if you are not currently experiencing any anxiety, it will help manage or prepare you for any upcoming events, as well as provide many other benefits. There are specific poses and breathing techniques that help specifically with anxiety and trauma. I recommend trying a class to benefit from the instructor's posture corrections. Also, many instructors will challenge your mind and keep bringing you back to the moment when you find that your mind is struggling and your thoughts wandering. There is some tranquility in the environment of many yoga studios that may provide practitioners with an oasis. Alternatively, there are videos, books, online videos, and websites dedicated to strengthening your practice.

Think it is too girly? Yoga is now in the athletic development programs for professional sports teams in sports such as hockey and snowboarding. I recently had the pleasure of working with trainers and an NHL team, and those guys know how much the strength, balance, flexibility, and mental stability of yoga can improve their game, prevent injuries, and give them an edge.

Namaste.

The Vicious Cycle of Emotional Eating

Glori's description of overeating to be bigger with the hope of avoiding unwanted sexual advances is not uncommon in women who have experienced sexual abuse.[3] The term "emotional eating" describes the practice of using food as a coping mechanism for dealing with stress. While the root cause or stressor is individual, many of us do engage in emotional eating. There is a complex relationship between food and emotions that stems from a stimulation of chemical pathways in the brain upon eating. This relationship makes emotional eating a very common issue—we have conditioned ourselves to eat in order to feel better. You might even be surprised to learn that you are an emotional eater (many if not most of us are). Let's discover how to identify emotional eating habits and look at tips for dealing with it to avoid excess intake/weight gain.

Registered psychologist Michelle Emmerling, MEd, offers this:

One way to conceptualize [emotional eating is] like an iceberg; we really only see the tip of it (the eating and weight related behaviours) and the real root causes that make up the majority of its substance are submerged under-neath. There we find struggles with sense of self, identity, difficulties with emotions, and overwhelming emotions like shame, fear, worthlessness, isolation, struggles with important relationships, jobs. Looking at it this way, food (or the visible behaviour we see) becomes a coping mechanism that helps the individual to distract from or avoid the real underlying issues that are deemed to be too overwhelming or threatening to handle. So if we focus on treating the weight and food related concerns only, we get lost on the path to recovery by losing sight of what the real struggles are, which is one reason that we see such a high rate of relapse or diet failures; we are looking for solutions in the wrong places. By focusing on weight or food related to "feeling fat," the individual has something concrete and tangible to focus on and the real problems that he or she is facing seem to disappear, but this is only a temporary relief. In order to heal and move through recovery from emotional eating, the key is to plunge beneath the surface and to work through the underlying concerns. It is only then that we can truly break free from food and weight concerns and live a wholehearted and content life.

Emotional eating is common among both men and women. Although the root cause of emotional eating may be different for each individual, the result is a developed physiological reliance on comfort foods, which can lead to unhealthy weight gain.

Unhappiness about your physical appearance can then further promote emotional eating, creating a vicious cycle. If you are experiencing emotional eating patterns, know that you are not alone. It is actually a biological response to stress that is rooted deep within our brains. Research shows that eating certain types of foods, particularly fatty foods, actually elicits a neurological reward response from the areas of our brains that control emotions. It's no wonder that we develop emotional eating habits! Fortunately, there are a number of techniques that can help to break the cycle of emotional eating. It is first important to identify the motivation for emotional eating: are you anxious, depressed, or simply bored?

Keeping a food diary for even just a few days can help you to begin to identify patterns of emotional eating. Write down the time of day, what you eat, how much of each food you've eaten, your hunger level on a scale of 1 to 5, and how you're feeling emotionally at the time of eating. This diary can be an effective tool to help reveal any patterns or connections between your emotional state and the amount or type of food you're choosing.

Once you have identified emotional eating, it is much easier to implement techniques to curb your cravings. If you have realized that a particularly stressful situation is contributing to emotional eating, try taking a break from what you're doing and perform a stress management technique such as meditation, deep breathing, stretching, or yoga. Perhaps you have identified that you tend to eat when bored: find ways to relieve your boredom that do not involve food. Some examples are to take a walk, exercise, read a book, or call a friend. If you find that you tend to eat foods high in fat or sugar when you eat emotionally, reduce the availability of these foods at home or work. Avoid purchasing these items while grocery shopping so that you don't have easy access to them. Don't keep extra cash or change around for vending machines at work, and bring healthy items such as fruit to snack on when you truly are hungry between meals at the office.

If the root of emotional eating is a serious issue, such as a history of abuse, depression, or uncontrolled anxiety, consider therapeutic help from a mental health professional. Identifying and dealing with the root of your emotions can help you avoid turning to food for comfort.

Resources

Local yoga classes—Try an online search, checking out local gyms, or ask in a yoga/athletic clothing store if they can point you in the right direction. You may want to try several different kinds of yoga and different instructors to find one you enjoy and that challenges you. Many yoga studios offer beginner classes that are a great place to start.

References

1. Speed-Andrews, AE et al. Predictors of adherence to an Iyengar yoga program in breast cancer survivors. *Int J Yoga*. 2012 Jan; 5(1):3-9.

2. Sparrowe, L. "Transcending Trauma." *Yoga International* (Fall 2011). Available online at: www.yogainternational.com.

3. Rohde, P et al. Associations of child sexual and physical abuse with obesity and depression in middle-aged women. *Child Abuse Negl*. 2008, 32(9):878-87.

Chapter 7

Training for a Cause

"'Look after yourself' means staying healthy, both in mind and body. To stay healthy, two things are key: exercise and a good diet. It's up to you to make good choices, and when you do, you can 'look after one another.' We're very lucky to have the things we have in Canada. Many are not so fortunate. We can all make a difference. Find your passion and follow it." — Martin Parnell

Martin Parnell's story is a wonderful example of the power that exists within each of us to create a better world for those around us through sheer determination and good will. Martin began running at the age of 47 and hasn't stopped since. Beginning with a 5K race, he has worked his way up to marathons, ultra-marathons, and Ironman events in support of a worthy and wonderful cause. While you may not go on to run a marathon, we hope that Martin's story and the information shared in this chapter will inspire you to get active and support a cause that's dear to your own heart in some way. Following Martin's story, we will provide you with important information on nutrition and physical activity if you are considering incorporating sport or challenging exercise into your life.

The Marathon Man: Martin's Story

I am passionate about helping children reach their full potential. I look at the world as a global village. It doesn't matter to me whether the child is at a local school in Cochrane, a First Nation community in northern Ontario, or a village in Benin, West Africa.

My journey started one evening in December 2002, when my younger brother Peter called me with a challenge. He and my other brother Andrew wanted to run the Calgary marathon the following July. I immediately said yes and put down the phone. The only problem was that I didn't run. As a kid I had played lots of sports, including soccer and tennis, but I wasn't very good at any of them. As I got older I switched to squash and golf. Then, at the age of 47, I had to start training for a 42.2K race.

The day after the call, I put on my old trainers and ran one km out from my house and one km back. It was not good. But I figured if I could do that, then the next time I could run two km out and two km back. By the time of the race, I was ready and finished in 3hrs 50min 22sec. My running career had begun. Over the next couple of years, I completed several more marathons, including Boston. I then started to do triathlons and ultra-marathons.

I had always wanted to see Africa and couldn't think of a better way of doing it than on a bike. In January 2005, I joined a group of 27 cyclists in Cairo prepared to cycle through Africa to Cape Town. It would take us four months to cross ten countries and travel over 10,000 km.

One morning, I was riding through a small village in Ethiopia. To my left, I noticed two young boys playing table tennis. Jumping off my bike, without saying a word, I indicated that I would like to play. One of them gave me his bat. Within five minutes, 100 kids were around the table yelling and shouting. I must have looked strange with my spandex shorts and Maple Leafs shirt. I played for about 20 minutes, before having to wave goodbye.

This simple event made me realize the power of sport and play and how it brings people together, regardless of age, culture, language, or religion.

In February 2009, I was introduced to Right To Play by my friend Tom Healy. This charity is the leading international humanitarian development organization to use the transformative power of sport and play to build essential skills in children. Through their work, they are driving social change in communities affected by war, poverty, and disease. Right To Play creates safe places where children can learn. The program helps them foster the hope that is essential for them to envision and realize a better future.

Right To Play trains coaches to run sport and play programs in their local communities. These activities promote opportunities for development and encourage the learning of life and leadership skills in order to build stronger, more peaceful communities. They also focus on health education by supporting national health objectives, in particular HIV and AIDS prevention and awareness, and vaccination campaigns.

Tom and I formed a group of like-minded people and called ourselves "Kids-U-Can." During the rest of the year, we competed in a number of road, bike, and triathlon races and fundraised for the charity. By the end of the year, we had raised $10,000. It was in the summer of that year that the idea of running lots of marathons came into my head. After chatting with my wife, Sue, I put a plan together and on January 1, 2010, I started my first marathon. By December 31, I had run 250 marathons and raised $320,000 for the kids.

The majority of my marathons were run in the Cochrane/Calgary area. Each morning I would get up and have a good breakfast of Mini-Wheats, yogurt, berries, a banana, and milk. The first month and a half I would leave my house and run along the road in the foothills of the Rockies. Many of the marathons were along the Bow River pathways. Sixty of them were run at schools. At a school I would talk to the children at morning assembly about "Marathon Quest 250," then I would head outside and run 100 times around their soccer field. During the day, children would join me and run a few laps. Many times they gave me their pocket money to help the "other" children. I ran with over 12,000 children during the year.

I ran seven official marathons: Vancouver, Victoria, Regina, Red Deer, Calgary, Las Vegas, and Boston. My fastest marathon was number 188 in Victoria, where I ran 3hr 43min 43sec—a Boston qualifier. During the year, I ran 10,550 km. This is equivalent to running from Calgary to Boston, down to New York, across to Seattle, up to Vancouver, and back to Calgary. I took 12,978,650 steps and used 25 pairs of shoes. I had 122 starts below freezing, the coldest day being -41 °C and the warmest was 32 °C.

On marathon number 28, I injured my left leg and had to stop running for two and a half weeks. I then walked eight marathons before I could start running again. During 2010 and 2011 I had monthly blood tests. I also underwent extensive medical testing. I kept close tabs on my health during the year. I was burning 5,000 calories a day and in the first month I lost 6 lbs, so my nutritionist put me on a high-fat diet. I ate full-fat milk, cheese, yogurt, and ice cream. This helped stabilize my weight. I was concerned about my cholesterol levels, but during the year, they were the lowest they've ever been.

My resting heart rate was 50 at the start of the year and dropped to 45 by the end. My average running heart rate was 99. A recent bone analysis indicated that my bone density and strength are equivalent to a 25-year-old elite alpine skier, which certainly surprised me.

In April 2011, Netball Alberta asked me to participate in an exhibition game of netball. I had never played the game, but three of my sisters and my wife had, so I had a general idea of what it was about. The game is played in 70 countries around the world by 20 million participants, but is practically unknown in North America. Netball Alberta wanted to increase the awareness of the game and I was one of the "Celebrity Players" invited to join them. The media was there and the game was a lots of fun.

In June 2011, I visited the West African country of Benin to spend time with children for whom I had raised funds. I joined them in a number of RTP activities and was caught up in their enthusiasm. It struck me that they didn't want handouts; they wanted a helping hand and someone to pay them some attention. On the last day I was in Benin I ran with a children's running club. I asked them the name of their club, and after a few minutes a girl named Parfait came over to me and said "The Undefeatables." Returning from Africa I realized that Marathon Quest 250 was not the end but the beginning.

In August 2011, I decided a bold plan was needed. I established the Quests for Kids initiative, aiming to complete 10 Quests in 5 years (2010–2014) and raise $1 million for Right To Play. This will support 20,000 children and encourage people to live an active, healthy lifestyle.

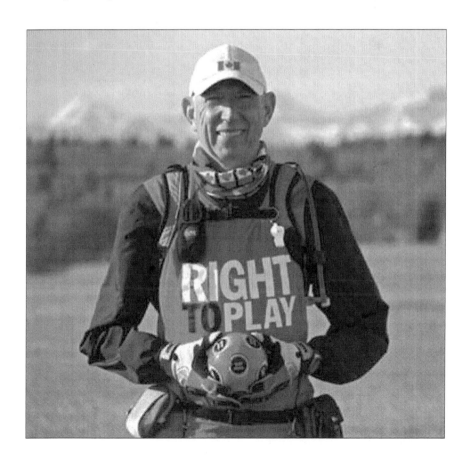

Criteria for a "Quest" are:

- The sport must be one that children can do at school or in the local community.
- Each "Quest" will be one of the following:
    1. An attempt to set or break the Guinness World Record for the longest time played in that sport in one continuous match or game.
    2. An attempt to set or break the Guinness World Record for the most players in an exhibition match or game of that sport.
    3. An extreme endurance event(s) in a sport.
- It will encourage children to become active and participate in sport.
- It will be a fundraiser for Right To Play.

I started thinking about the next fundraising event and the idea that it would be based on beating the Guinness World Record for an endurance sport came to mind. I checked with Guinness and found that the record for the longest game of netball played was 60 hours. The next day, I contacted a member of Netball Alberta, Julie Arnold, and put forward my idea. She was very enthusiastic and the planning process started.

So Netball Quest 61 became my second Quest. On September 16, 2011, two teams lined up at a recreational centre in Calgary and the game was on. The majority of the players were from the women's A and B leagues. However, there were several rookie players. Lau Mafuru had recently arrived from Tanzania. Lau operated a trekking company, Boma Africa, and had personally ascended Mount Kilimanjaro over 50 times. Buzz Bishop was a radio DJ, and breaking a Guinness World Record was on the top of his bucket list. Christina Smith was an Olympic bobsledder looking for an opportunity to help children.

At 6:30 am, Monday, September 19, 2011, this amazing team completed a total of 61 hours, breaking the Guinness World Record. A total of $22,600 was raised, allowing 452 children to participate in a Right To Play program.

The participants of this record-breaking event were sixteen women and eight men. The youngest was 17 and the oldest 55. Their countries of birth include Canada, England, Australia, New Zealand, Fiji, Tanzania, and South Africa. The majority of them had not been through such a physically and mentally gruelling ordeal before. Twenty-four players started and twenty-four finished. For many of them it was a life-changing experience.

In 2012, I plan to complete three more Quests. Quest Three was Lacrosse Quest 24, held in April 2012. A new Guinness World Record for indoor lacrosse was set at 24 hours and $35,000 was raised for RTP. I had never played lacrosse before, and it was a blast learning the game. Quest Four is Cook Islands Quest 100. In September, a group of 20 of us will head down to the Pacific Islands. The race around the island of Rarotonga is 32K; however, I plan to run 100 km—three times around the island plus a little bit more. We hope to raise $25,000 for RTP. Quest Five is Soccer Quest 42 in October. An attempt will be made to beat the record for the longest game of five-a-side soccer. The current record is 40 hours. We are aiming to complete 42 hours and raise $25,000 for RTP.

It's important to realize that you can make a difference. Right To Play has taught me a lot. Their motto is "Look after yourself, look after one another." Let's think about this. "Look after yourself" means staying healthy, both in mind and body. To stay healthy, two things are key: exercise and a good diet. It's up to you to make good choices, and when you do, you can "look after one another." We're very lucky to have the things we have in Canada. Many are not so fortunate. We can all make a difference.

Find your passion and follow it.

For more information on Martin Parnell and his Marathon Quest, visit: *www.marathonquest250.com.*

Sport Nutrition: Building Blocks for Training

If you're venturing on a physical quest, whether it be long-distance running such as Martin's marathons, cycling on the MS Bike Tour like Judy (Chapter 5), a triathlon, or the Tough Mudder obstacle race, it is obvious that planning your physical training so that your body can endure and excel at your event is of great importance. Of equal importance is planning your dietary intake to be sure that your body is appropriately fuelled for your training and events, whether competitive or recreational. Optimizing performance requires a balance of healthy eating, activity and training, and adequate rest.

If you are training for a specific event, you should follow a healthy and balanced diet most of the time prior to the event. It's important to note that training for an event is not the most appropriate time to attempt weight loss. Weight loss is inevitably a loss of both fat and muscle, and requires that you take in fewer calories than you burn. Eating too few calories during training leads to reduced endurance, compromised immune function, increased requirements for recovery time (and consequently increased risk for injury), and decreased strength/muscle mass. This becomes a problem, as training will increase your daily calorie requirements, so actively trying to lose weight by cutting calories and increasing activity will result in a less-than-optimal athletic performance as you train. Bottom line: If you are attempting to lose weight, this is best attempted in the off-season.

Which foods should you focus on while training?

- *Carbohydrates*—Much to the chagrin of low-carb dieters every-where, those engaging in regular physical activity and/or athletic training should ensure adequate carbohydrate intake. Carbohydrates give our bodies the basic sugars needed for energy (simple sugars are the primary source of fuel for both the body and brain). Physiologically speaking, the body's preferred source of energy is glucose. The body will break down more complex carbohydrates in the digestive process to obtain this simple sugar for fuel. Glucose is stored in the body's muscles and liver as glycogen, which is broken down by the body for energy and is especially important during endurance activities. Choosing six to seven servings of grains, seven to eight servings of fruit or vegetables, and two to three servings of milk and dairy alternatives daily will provide you with adequate carbohydrates and help to build your glycogen stores for endurance activities. As your energy needs increase with increased training time, use your hunger as a gauge to bring up your intake from all healthy food sources to maintain a balanced diet.

- *Protein*—Protein from food is used by the body to build and replenish our skin, nails, hair, and muscle and is also an important factor in our immune systems. Protein, whether obtained from ingesting food sources or depleted from our muscle stores, is used as an energy source by the body when inadequate carbohydrates are consumed. Over time, protein taken from the muscles reduces muscle mass and impairs athletic performance. Aim to eat a protein source at each meal, and for those with high calorie needs, also at each snack. Some examples of good protein choices are lean meats, fish, poultry, nuts, tofu, eggs, legumes, and hummus. It is a performance mistake to overload on protein and eat fewer carbohydrates; inadequate carbohydrate intake will hinder muscle-building capacity. Overloading can also lead to dehydration and calcium losses in the body.

- *Fluids*—Inadequate water intake will severely inhibit athletic performance and endurance. Thirst is actually a late signal of dehydration; by the time you feel thirsty, you've already lost 1 to 2 percent of your body's hydration status (a number that is associated with reduced athletic capacity and performance). Dehydration cannot be cured *during* exercise, so prevention is crucial! Remember to consider your environment: heat and humidity both increase your fluid requirements. Plain cool water is recommended for activity less than one hour in duration, and sports drinks (which contain carbohydrates, fluid, and electrolytes) are optimized to maintain athletic performance for activities longer than one hour. It is important to note that diluting sports drinks with too much water makes their contents insignificant for sport performance; if you have difficulty tolerating them, try an easily digested snack or sports gel and follow with water. Caffeinated energy drinks, such as Red Bull, are not recommended for activity, as they can promote dehydration and result in cramping. Your nutrition during training is important to fuel your physical needs and optimize performance, but it also allows your body to get used to the foods or drinks you will be using during the main event. Read more about the importance of hydration on page 97.

Event-Day Nutrition: Do's and Don't's

If you have properly fuelled your body in the weeks or months leading up to an event, you have set yourself up for success. What you eat on the day of your event (prior to, during, and following your event) will make an immediate and direct impact on your physical performance. Eating properly on the day of your event helps to enhance endurance performance by providing an available source of energy, prevent hunger during the event, enhance mental alertness, ensure adequate hydration, and promote recovery. Both the foods you choose and the timing of your intake are critical.

Timing

• Eat two to four hours before the start of your event to allow sufficient time for food to clear your stomach.

• Consuming a source of carbohydrates throughout your event can help with endurance activities.

• Eating after the event can promote recovery and restore your body's reserve of glycogen (the storage form of glucose in your body). Consume a carbohydrate-rich food within 15 minutes of finishing the activity and replenish further with a full meal within 2 hours.

Food Choices

Your pre-event meal should be high in complex carbohydrates, moderate in protein, low in fat, and include a source of fluids. This will allow for a rate of digestion that ensures food is cleared from the stomach by the beginning of your event. A higher-fat meal can prolong the length of time that food takes to clear the stomach, which will make for an uncomfortable event and poor availability of energy for activity. Other performance-hindering culprits to limit or avoid on the date of your event include alcohol, salt, and caffeine. (Moderate caffeine is okay if it is your usual routine, but don't try adding caffeine on the day of the event if your system is not used to it.)

Some examples of good pre-event meals include:

• Cereal with low-fat milk (or a fluid milk alternative such as a fortified soy/rice beverage), banana, 1.5 to 2 cups of water.

• Muffin, yogurt, orange, 2 cups of water.

- Turkey sandwich on whole wheat bread, apple, 2 cups of water.
- Rolled oats, a peach, scrambled eggs, 1 cup of milk/fluid milk alternative, 1 cup of water.

The golden rule with respect to pre-event eating is to *never try foods on the date of the event that you have not tested in training*. If possible, schedule at least a few training sessions prior to the event that are performed at the same time of day at which your event is scheduled; this will provide you with opportunities to test out your pre-event meal. This testing allows you to determine how far in advance to eat and how much to eat in order to feel satisfied but not still full when your event begins. It will help you gauge how the foods make you feel during the activity. The "right" meal is very individual, so be sure to try it out in advance.

As noted above, consuming a source of carbohydrates along with fluids throughout your event can improve endurance and prevent hunger in events longer than one hour in duration. General recommendations are to take in 30 to 60 g of carbohydrates per hour: this is equivalent to about two cups of a sports drink (not the "low calorie" versions), one or two sports gels, half a cup of fresh fruit, a quarter cup of dried fruit, or half a bagel. Test out which works best for you in advance throughout your training.

Finally, recovery eating serves to restore your body's energy reserves. Within 15 minutes of completing your event, take in a carbohydrate source such as juice, fruit, milk, yogurt, or a muffin. Then further replenish within two hours post-event with another 50 g of carbohydrates (e.g., a muffin or bagel and a piece of fruit). Remember to rehydrate with at least two cups of fluid for every pound of water weight lost (non-alcoholic decaffeinated beverages are best for hydration).

Nutrition works in harmony with proper training and adequate rest throughout your training or activity, and can help maximize performance on the date of an athletic event. Don't shortchange your training efforts with suboptimal nutrition!

Injury Prevention During Exercise

Injury prevention is critical. Let's face it, if you are injured you will probably no longer exercise (at least for a while). Depending on the injury, it may affect the activities of daily living, such as walking, carrying grocery bags, or driving.

Don't get me wrong, fear of injury should not be a deterrent from exercise. I assure you the damage being done by sitting is much worse than exercise. When looking at the pros and cons, doing exercise always wins. However, there are some things you can do to lower your risk of injury.

Check with Your Doc

If you are new to exercising, especially if over the age of 40 for men and 50 for women, or have any concerns whatsoever, see your physician. Your physician should be thrilled you are beginning a lifestyle change and will do a checkup to make sure you are good to go.

Know the signs of caution. Stop exercising if you experience any of the following:

- Chest Pain or Discomfort
  - **What**: Uncomfortable feelings of pressure, pain, squeezing, or heaviness.
  - **Where**: In the centre of the chest, spread through the front of the chest, or radiating to the shoulder(s), arm(s), neck, and back.
  - **What to Do**: Stop, sit, or lie down. If it does not stop after two to four minutes, go to the emergency room. If it goes away, go to the doctor.

- Severe Nausea, Shortness of Breath, Sweating, or Feeling Light-headed—Call your doctor.

If exercising outside, try to always exercise with a partner or let someone know where you are going.

Gradually Increase Over Time

Going from zero to full speed in ten seconds is only cool in a sports car; your body, however, needs time to adapt. Whatever exercise you choose, it is important to work up slowly. Start with very light weight or intensity and build up over time. It is very important for your muscles and your heart to adapt to the load you are putting on them.

Muscle is formed by microscopic tears that result from exercise; your body then repairs these tears, making the muscle stronger. You want to find the balance of forming enough tears so the muscle strengthens but not too many that it cannot heal quickly. It is normal to experience mild delayed onset muscle soreness (DOMS) a day or two after a workout, but it should never result in pain or the inability to move.

Keeping track of your workouts (see Chapter 5) can help you progress appropriately. If you take time off of exercise for whatever reason, remember not to jump back into exercise where you left off. Go back a couple of steps, and again, start slowly.

Form

Incorrect form is one of the biggest reasons for injury during exercise. Whatever activity you decide to take part in, make sure proper form is at the top of your list of priorities. Form is much more important than the weight you are lifting. Form first, form first, form first!

Seek help from experts in the field. If you are lifting weights at a gym, for example, and would like to ensure you are performing a lift with the proper technique, ask a trainer. Look in the mirror as they guide you through the exercise, so you can replicate the same movement.

Walking and running is an activity that is often performed incorrectly. It is much easier to explain proper form with visuals, so on *inspiremewell.com* we have provided videos and pictures to adequately describe these activities.

Warm Up and Cool Down

Warm Up

Warming up before exercise for about five to ten minutes in an activity similar to the activity you are about to engage in increases your muscles' ability to contract and relax quickly. A proper warm up also increases muscle elasticity, decreasing the risk of strains and pulls. Gradually warming up reduces the stress on the heart, increases blood flow to the working muscles, and improves the range of motion around a joint. For example, if you are going for a jog, warm up by walking and then slowly work up to a jog.

Cool Down

Cooling down simply means slowing down (not stopping completely) after exercise. When you continue to move around after exercise, at a very low intensity for five to ten minutes, it helps your blood pressure and heart rate return to resting levels. For example, after your jog, slow down or walk to cool down. It also protects your muscles from injuries and may reduce muscles stiffness. After your cool down is the ideal time to stretch out your muscles, as they will still be warm.

Develop a Drinking Problem

Water is the most important nutrient for life. It is vital for body temperature regulation, blood pressure stabilization, transportation of nutrients, joint lubrication, and so much more. It becomes even more important when you are exercising. The longer and the more intensely you are exercising, the more important hydration becomes for comfort, performance, and safety.

Dehydration

Risks of dehydration are serious. When you are dehydrated, it becomes increasingly difficult to circulate blood and for the body to function, which may also lead to muscle cramps, dizziness, fatigue, and heat illness, including heat exhaustion and heat stroke.

Common causes of dehydration during exercise:
- Not drinking enough
- Excessive sweating
- Not replacing fluid losses during and after exercise
- Exercising in dry hot weather
- Drinking only when thirsty (you are already dehydrated when you are thirsty)

Your Hydration Needs

Everyone sweats, intakes water, and retains water differently. It is impossible to determine the exact amount someone should drink, but there are guidelines you can follow.

The American College of Sports Medicine suggests that:

individuals should develop customized fluid replacement programs that prevent excessive (greater than 2 percent body weight reductions from baseline body weight) dehydration. The routine measurement of pre- and post-exercise body weights is useful for determining sweat rates and customized fluid replacement programs. Consumption of beverages containing electrolytes and carbohydrates can help sustain fluid-electrolyte balance and exercise performance.[1]

To review, general guidelines for hydration during activity include:

Before exercise:
- Drink about two cups of water, two to three hours before exercise
- Drink one cup 10 to 15 minutes before exercise

During exercise:
- Drink one cup every 10 to 15 minutes during exercise
- If exercising longer than an hour, drink one cup of a sports

drink every 15 to 30 minutes

After exercise:

- Weigh yourself before and after exercise and replace fluid losses
- Drink two cups water for every pound lost
- Consume something to replenish your carbohydrates and protein within two hours after exercise to replenish glycogen stores

Listen to Your Body

I saw a guy at the gym. You know the type—huge muscles, no neck? He had a shirt on that said, "Pain is simply weakness leaving the body." This statement is incorrect. Although there is a certain amount of fatigue or discomfort you can push through, pain is telling you that something is wrong and it is a way of preventing further damage.

If something hurts during or after exercise, to the point that you are concerned, go to a physician or physiotherapist to address your concerns. It may be a matter of changing form during your exercise, resting, or you may need some rehabilitation.

Rest and Recovery

If you are Type A personality like me, this can be the most difficult aspect of exercise. Rest and recovery should always be factored into a strength and conditioning program, as it is just as important as the program design itself. Too much exercise can cause an increase in levels of the stress hormones and minimizes or stops strength gains. This is where the importance of restoration and recovery come into play.

Sleep, a variety of activities, and days off are essential to any exercise program. Not taking enough rest between bouts of exercise can result in poorer fitness gains and injury in the long run. The amount of rest is dependent on the training intensity and the types of activities you are performing. Cardio can be performed daily; however, the intensity and type should be varied. You should take at least a day off between strength training sessions.

Cross-Train

Adding a variety of exercises to your routine relieves the boredom of your workout and is key to a well-rounded exercise regime. For example, if you bike three times a week at the same pace for the same duration or distance, your program will get very boring and it will actually decrease your fitness because your muscles and heart are no longer being challenged.

Try to incorporate at least two different types of aerobic physical activities and a variety of strength training in your weekly routine to improve your overall aerobic capacity, build overall muscle strength, and reduce the chance of an overuse injury. Here are some benefits of a variety of activities:

- It's less boring!
- It allows you to be flexible about your training needs and plans. For example, if your bike is getting repaired, you can go for a swim or run instead.
- It creates better all-around conditioning and incorporates different muscle groups.
- It reduces the risk of injury.
- You can continue to train while injured. For example, if you have a knee injury, perhaps a swim may be a better option than running or biking.
- It improves the condition of the minor muscles that support the major muscle groups and can help your skill, agility, and balance.

What exercises could make up a good cross-training routine? Consider activities you enjoy!

Cardiovascular exercise:
- Running
- Swimming
- Cycling
- Rowing
- Climbing stairs
- Jumping rope
- Skating (inline or ice)
- Skiing (cross-country or downhill)
- Squash/basketball/soccer and so many other sports

Strength training exercises:
- Weightlifting
- Using bands
- Calisthenics (push-ups, crunches, pull-ups)
- Pilates

Other things to consider:
- Flexibility (stretching, yoga)
- Speed, agility, and balance drills (sport specific or not)
- Circuit training, sprinting, and other forms of skill conditioning

Adding a variety of activities allows you to mix and match your activities to suit your training needs, interests, and schedule. The variety allows you to see even more benefits from exercise than a single activity program. Get started now!

Dress Properly

Your Shoes

Shoes are the most important piece of equipment for exercise, especially running or walking. A good pair of shoes can provide support and cushioning and can help prevent injuries; therefore, it is important to identify good shoes for your foot. Before deciding on a good shoe, it helps to know your own foot—is your arch low, medium, or high? It is easy to assess what type of arch you have, just wet the bottom of your foot and step on a hard surface. If the forefoot and heel areas are connected by a thin line, you have high-arched feet. If the footprint looks like the shape of your foot, you have a low arch. A medium arch will fall somewhere in between.

If you have high arches, your foot will not be very flexible and you will want a cushioned shoe. If you are flatfooted or have low arches, your feet will be too flexible and you will need a motion-controlled shoe. If you have a medium arch, you should request a stability shoe.

The type of exercise is important to consider when shopping for shoes. Let the sales associate at the store know if you are looking for a walking, running (forward motion shoe), or cross-trainer (forward *and* side-to-side motion).

Most stores that sell athletic shoes will have trained staff who are knowledgeable about the different kinds of shoes. It is useful to them if you bring an old pair of runners so that they can see the pattern of wear on the soles of the shoes.

Shoe buying tips:
- Shop late in the day because your feel swell as the days go on.
- Measure your foot while standing.
- Try both your shoes on with the socks you wear during exercise. (If you have orthotics, bring them.)
- Buy for your larger foot. (Feet are rarely the exact same size.)
- Allow a thumbnail's width between the shoe and your big toe.
- Choose a shoe that is comfortable right away.
- Shoes should feel good around the ball of your foot, through the arch, and fit snuggly at the heel.
- Wear your shoes around the house before you use them for exercise, and run or walk on a treadmill. Return them if there is a problem.

Shop around! As noted above, many stores that specialize in running or walking shoes will have experts there to help make your decision easier.

Happy shopping!

Your Skin

Wear sunscreen! And not just any sunscreen; dermatologists are now recommending an SPF of over 30. If you are planning water activities, your sunscreen needs to be waterproof, and when you get out of the water, dry off and reapply. If you are engaging in land-based exercise, wear sweat-proof sunscreen and reapply often, especially after your activity.

Many athletic companies are now making athletic clothing specific for exercising in the heat that is lightweight and takes the sweat off your body with SPF built in.

NOTE: Sunburns prior to the age of 18 double your risk of skin cancer. Make sure you protect your children's skin![2]

Your Body

Wear shorts, T-shirts, or workout pants to exercise. You should be comfortable. You should wear clothing that is breathable, cool, and that will allow you to move unrestricted. There are a number of fabrics on the market that will wick moisture away from your body and allow the fabric to dry faster, therefore preventing chafing and blisters. Fabrics such as Coolmax and polypropylene are commonly used in today's exercise fashions. Make sure that clothing such as socks and sports bras fit well. These items should be snug and made from a breathable moisture-wicking material.

Dressing for the seasons: When exercising outside, it is important to remember that the weather can change quickly, so you need to be prepared. Before exercising outdoors, remember to check the weather and to wear sunglasses and sunscreen. Select clothing made from breathable material; cotton can be heavy when wet and

104 — Inspire Me Well

cause chafing. In the winter, layering is very important. The layer closest to the skin should be close fitting and made of a moisture-wicking material. The next layer should be an insulating layer, such as fleece or wool. The last layer should be wind and water resistant. Remember to keep your hands and feet covered and to wear a hat, since 50 percent of the body's heat is lost through the head. If the wind chill has dropped below -20 °C, you should exercise indoors…or wait for a while, since the weather can change quickly in Canada!

References

1. Swaka, MN et al. Exercise and fluid replacement. *Medicine & Science in Sports & Exercise*. 2007, 39 (2) pp. 377–90.

2. Skin Cancer Foundation. (2012). "Facts about Sunburn and Skin Cancer." Available online at: www.skincancer.org/prevention/sunburn/facts-about-sunburn-and-skin-cancer.

Chapter 8

Coping with Cancer

"My mom always told me to take care of my body, as it is the only one you get." — Ashley Rose

Cancer. This small word has so many meanings to each of us. It is a horrific disease that can be the fight of a lifetime. It is the source of pain, suffering, sorrow, and controversy, but it can also bring out the best in humankind. Ashley shares her cancer experience and how she was influenced by behaviours she could take control of: exercise and nutrition. Researchers are now investigating the role lifestyle behaviours such as exercise and nutrition have on the complete spectrum of the disease from prevention to survivorship. After Ashley's story we highlight some of the ground-breaking research being done in this area.

Ashley's Story

I can honestly say that now, at the age of 28, I am the most active and healthiest I have ever been. Growing up as the oldest child of four, I remember how fitness and healthy living was always instilled in us kids. My dad was a talented athlete growing up, especially in hockey, baseball, and handball (where he made it to the national level before blowing out his knee!). He was always the coach on our various sports teams, whether it was hockey, soccer, or fastball. All of my siblings and I started playing organized sports at the age of four, and that love for sports carried on into our adulthood. My sisters and I also danced, which is a great way for young girls to keep active and improve balance and coordination skills!

Our mom always made sure that we stayed active and ate healthily. Feeding a family of six is not cheap, but that never meant that our health suffered. In fact, as kids we thought that Pop-Tarts only came out in the summer because the only time they were allowed was when we were going on camping trips! My mom always made sure there was a fresh, homemade, healthy (and often organic) meal on the table for us, even though she worked evenings and weekends around my dad's schedule to make sure that there was always a parent at home. I learned to appreciate these meals even more in university; nothing beats coming home from class and grabbing homemade soup and buns for dinner before settling in for a long night of studying ahead.

As a teenager, I struggled with weight and body issues, as most girls do. While I love my Ukrainian heritage, I am still learning to love the curves that come with that. My mom always told me to take care of my body, as it is the only one you get. This thinking was especially helpful in my teenage years when I was learning not only to love my body, but also to treat it right.

When I was 21 and in my fourth year of university, I was diagnosed with thyroid cancer.

The thyroid is known as the "master gland"—the one that controls hormones and metabolism. The first course of action was to remove the thyroid, then a course of radioactive iodine, or RAI, which is a sort of oral chemotherapy that targets the cancerous thyroid cells and kills off any remaining thyroid tissue. After my initial surgery, because the cancer had spread into surrounding lymph nodes and muscle tissue, another surgery was planned, followed by two or three more RAI treatments.

Around the time of my diagnosis, I had struggled to understand why I was putting on weight, but in hindsight I realize that it was due to the issues with my thyroid. From the time my thyroid was removed in 2004, it took nearly two years to determine the correct dosage of synthetic thyroid hormone for my body. TWO YEARS! Throughout that time, of course, my weight fluctuated as did my size. I was anywhere from a size 4 to 12. I actually worked part-time at The Gap in part so that I could afford pants in every size.

I had friends who were obsessing about the latest fad diets, or commenting on how their clothes didn't fit right anymore (and I had to laugh to myself, as I could not tell it was because they had gained or lost those ten pounds). For me, while my weight continued to fluctuate, I was just happy to have four functioning limbs and a body that was on the road to recovery. I was focused on the fight of my life—overcoming cancer.

RAI treatment works on the theory that only thyroid tissue and thyroid cancer cells absorb the radioactive iodine. By injecting radioactive iodine into the body, the body is so depleted of iodine that if any remnant thyroid tissue or cancer cells are remaining, they show up very easily on the scan. The progression of the cancer is measured by looking at the "uptake" of the iodine.

After my first RAI treatment, I focused a lot on healthy eating. Due to having staples and a drain in my neck, it helped that I could not chew a lot, so many antioxidant-containing smoothies were consumed! I also did a lot of energy work, such as meditation, reiki, visualization, craniosacral treatments, and acupuncture. Taking an active approach to my health not only felt good physically, but mentally too. I was regaining power and ownership over my body.

I remember my mom telling me to visualize little Pac-Men (from the video game) eating up my cancer. At the time I rolled my eyes at her, but behind closed doors I tried it because I figured, what did I have to lose?

Following my first surgery and RAI treatment, we walked into the oncologist's office expecting to hear of another surgery date, as had been previously discussed. Amazingly, he indicated that he was pleased with how well I had responded to the RAI. Rather than schedule another surgery, he wanted to see if another dosage of it would kill off the remaining cancer cells. He anticipated possibly two more RAI treatments.

As challenging as it is not to have a thyroid, the preparation for RAI treatments can be just as challenging. There is a 40-day protocol to follow, which involves being off of synthetic thyroid hormone for that time (so no metabolism regulation in your body) and following a strict low-iodine diet so that when the patient ingests the radioactive iodine, the cancerous cells are so starved for iodine that they quickly and readily absorb it. The week before the scheduled RAI treatment, a tracer dosage of RAI is injected, followed by two or three scans to determine the uptake and amount of cancerous cells.

You really do not realize just how many foods have iodine in them! I could not eat out during that time. I ate only healthy, fresh, organic foods. Did you know that cows' teats are wiped with iodized cloths? This meant that I couldn't have milk, butter, or chocolate on the diet. Beans or legumes soak up iodine in the soil, so those were also a no-no. So was red dye, meat, tap water, and anything canned or packaged in metallic containers (again, iodine can be leached into food). Some thyroid cancer patients go as far as to call it "hypo hell," although I actually felt really good on the diet; I was not putting anymore synthetic hormone in my body and was eating only fresh natural foods. (I didn't escape "side effect free" though. I encountered fainting spells, sluggishness, and hair loss, just to name a few side effects.)

I went through the 40-day protocol, and sat in the waiting room of the cancer hospital, preparing to be admitted for another RAI treatment. Hospitalization was required due to high levels of radioactivity I was emitting. Any waste had to be double wrapped and kept in a shed for the half-life of the radiation. I couldn't go near children or seniors for weeks. I had to be away from family. I had to wear two pair of socks (so when I walked I wasn't leaving traces) and wipe down every surface I touched. I had to flush three times after using the washroom and suck on sour candies so that my salivary glands would not succumb to the RAI. I also had to shower at least twice daily to wash the RAI from my body, and express my eyes with warm water so that my tear ducts would not be affected. Unfortunately, my tear ducts were affected. It was a nasty side effect that lasted three years post-treatment. Imagine feeling like you have sand in your eyes all the time!

A surprising thing happened when I went to my oncologist's office for my second RAI treatment. I am not sure why, how, or what happened, but when I walked in he looked at me and said: "Go home." My parents and I just looked at each other in disbelief. He said my scans came back clean. No evidence of cancer. No more RAI. No more surgeries. We hugged. We cried. We high-fived. Then we went to Tim Hortons!

While it has been seven years since I heard I had cancer, a reoccurrence with this type of cancer, especially five or ten years post-diagnosis is a very real possibility. Unfortunately, so is the chance of developing a secondary cancer, especially breast and ovarian cancer, because they, along with my thyroid, also absorbed the RAI.

I have learned to embrace the moment and take nothing for granted. You never know when you may not get that moment back. However, the fact that I can control what goes in my body, how I manage stress, and how I choose to live provides me with great strength and a belief that I hopefully will never have to experience cancer again.

I feel so empowered that I can elevate my mood and change my appearance by controlling what goes in my body. By eating healthily, continuing daily runs, and staying active, I have maintained a healthy weight that I am happy about for the past two years. I no longer weigh myself. I determine if I've changed weight by counting how many lunges I need to do to fit into my skinny jeans.

I still maintain an active healthy lifestyle. Just last summer I was fortunate to go on a kayaking expedition with eight other female cancer survivors from all over the country. We lived on the river for nine days and kayaked over 80 km. It was exhilarating, breathtaking, and life-changing!

Now I take time to smell the roses, have spontaneous adventures, be silly and laugh, and enjoy every precious moment because it just feels so much sweeter. And I always make room for dessert (in moderation, of course) because life is just too short!

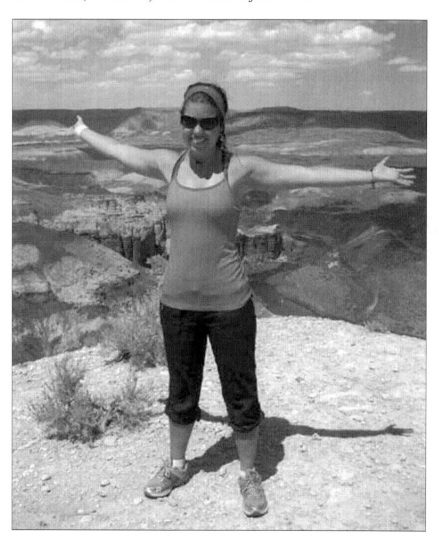

Exercise and Cancer

When many people think about the link between exercise and cancer, they think of the runs or walks in support for research of particular diseases (Run for the Cure, Underwear Affair, Team in Training). Many people do not know that exercise has a direct protective effect against some kinds of cancer. I am NOT saying it will completely take away someone's chances of having the disease, but it *will reduce the risk* of the disease, and for cancer survivors it will reduce the risk of recurrence, increase quality of life, help with weight management, and improve physical function and mental well-being (among many other positive side effects). In a report by the World Cancer Research Fund titled *Food, Nutrition, Physical Activity and the Prevention of Cancer: A Global Perspective*,[1] it is estimated that one third of cancers can be prevented through lifestyle changes such as increased physical activity, improved nutrition, and reduction of body fat.

How Exactly Does Exercise Protect Against Cancer?

The exact mechanism of how exercise prevents cancer is not well understood. More research is required to determine what exactly happens in the body. There are several systems in the body through which exercise might exert a protective effect against cancer; however, it is probably a combination of several biological mechanisms. Exercise alters the body's energy balance, hormone levels, metabolism, and insulin growth factor. The shift in each of these mechanisms has been shown to reduce the risk of cancer. The change with the greatest cancer protective effects is the positive influence exercise has on your immune system and inflammatory response.

Still not sold on the idea that moving every day can help prevent cancer? Check out the evidence:

Colon—There have been over 50 studies performed examining

the protective effects of exercise and colon cancer. The results indicate that adults who increase either the intensity or duration of their exercise decreased their colon cancer risk by 30 to 40 percent! This is compared to inactive people performing less than 150 minutes of moderate activity a week and is independent of body fat. These studies also indicated the greatest risk reductions were in people who were more active.

There are also studies that look at exercise after colon cancer, so regardless of a person's activity level before a colon cancer diagnosis, increasing exercise post-treatment will reduce their chances of the colon cancer returning by up to 50 percent.[2] We currently cannot offer any drug or other behaviour that has an impact as significant as exercise on disease-free survivorship.

Breast—There are over 60 studies examining the link between exercise and breast cancer. The effect of exercise on breast cancer prevention range from 20 to 80 percent (depending on factors such as the age or race of the women studied). Increasing exercise at any time in a woman's life has a protective effect, even in adolescence.

Although less research has been done on endometrial, prostate, and lung cancers, preliminary studies show exercise has a protective effect against these cancers.[3]

The minimum amount of exercise needed to benefit from these protective effects is 150 minutes per week of moderate intensity activity (such as brisk walking, doubles tennis, or recreational swimming) OR 75 minutes of vigorous activity (such as jogging/running, playing soccer, singles tennis, or swimming laps). Protective effects were greater for those who did more activity than the base recommendations. Many studies are suggesting 30 to 60 minutes of moderate activity every day.

SIDE NOTE: Moderate exercise is when your heart rate is elevated, you are sweating lightly, and are breathing heavier than normal. If you can keep up a conversation but cannot sing while you are working out, you are working at moderate intensity. If you cannot sing (physically unable to catch your breath to do so, not because you're tone deaf), you are working at a vigorous intensity.

These findings are all independent of body fat, so if you are also reducing your body fat and increasing muscle mass through exercise and your nutritional intake, you are further increasing the protective effects and protecting yourself from cancer. Think about how exciting this is: We have the power to reduce our chances of getting cancer with such simple day-to-day choices.

Exercise During and After Cancer Treatments

Exercise has extensive benefits for cancer survivors, even if they have never been active before. This research is advancing in leaps and bounds to encompass survivors of all different kinds of cancer, from all around the world. This is my area of study, so please excuse the enthusiasm on the subject.

Cancer survivorship is defined from the moment of diagnosis to the end of life. Studies of the effects of exercise on cancer have been done on many stages of the cancer continuum such as pre-treatment, during treatment, post-treatment, and long-term survivorship. Here are some examples of the cutting-edge research in this field.

Based on reviews of all the studies done on cancer survivors during treatment, it has been concluded that exercise is not only safe and feasible during cancer treatments, but it may also improve physical functioning, decrease fatigue, and positively influence many aspects of quality of life. The recommendations for people undergoing cancer treatment are to maintain exercise as much as possible. If you have been inactive before treatment, it is recommended to engage in low intensity exercise (i.e., slow walks, stretching, yoga) and build up slowly.[4]

One very exciting finding was an increased chemotherapy completion rate in breast cancer survivors. In this study, breast cancer survivors would come into a fitness centre for an aerobic workout or an aerobic workout plus weights three times a week during the length of their chemotherapy (usually for about three months).[5] At the beginning of the study, breast cancer survivors were divided into three groups: a resistance-training group, an aerobic group, and a usual care group. The usual care group did not receive any exercise training.

When patients are diagnosed with cancer, a treatment plan is made up. For example: six rounds of X drug, every three weeks. This plan can be interrupted by many circumstances, such as drug side effects or low white blood cell count. This study showed a significant positive effect of exercise on the women's ability to complete their treatment plans: 78 percent of those in the resistance-training group and 74.4 percent in the aerobic exercise group completed at least 85 percent of their recommended chemotherapy. In the control group receiving usual care, 65.9 percent completed at least 85 percent of their recommended chemotherapy prescription. Essentially, women in the exercise groups were given more of their drugs on time allowing them to benefit from their full chemotherapy dosage.

A very common complaint with cancer survivors after treatment is fatigue. This fatigue is so much more than "being tired." Everyone can be tired from time to time, after certain activities and at the end of the day, and we can usually resolve tiredness with a good night's sleep. Fatigue on the other hand is less cause and effect. There is not a particular event that causes fatigue, and it will not be resolved with sleep. Fatigue is full body lethargy and excessive tiredness that affects your daily living activities and diminishes quality of life.

For people suffering from cancer-related fatigue, exercise is one of the treatments that has demonstrated the most promise. I realize that it may seem counterintuitive, and that the natural response to fatigue is to rest. Margie McNeely and Kerry Courneya released a review of literature and physical activity guidelines for cancer survivors experiencing fatigue.[6] After treatment, it is recommended to return to activity as soon as possible. Just as for anyone starting to exercise again after a period of inactivity, it is important to start slowly and slowly build up to guidelines, to be discussed below. Cancer and cancer treatment side effects may remain for months, years, or indefinitely after treatment. Exercise may fit into your life differently than before cancer treatment. For example, if you have peripheral neuropathy, falling may be a new concern, so it may be easier and safer to ride a stationary bike instead of walking on a treadmill.

Studies in cancer survivors post-treatment have demonstrated many positive outcomes, including better quality of life, cardiovascular fitness, self-esteem, and lower anxiety and stress. There have also been studies demonstrating lower risk of cancer recurrence and improved overall mortality among breast, colorectal, prostate, and ovarian cancer survivors.

How Much Physical Activity Should Survivors Be Doing?

The American College of Sports Medicine has determined that exercise is safe and beneficial for cancer patients and survivors.[4] The exercise recommendations they put forward for cancer survivors indicate that survivors should be working their way up to 150 minutes of moderate exercise a week. The American Cancer Society provides the same guidelines. Some studies have shown a dose-response relationship: the more exercise you do, the more benefits you will receive. Remember though, it is important to build up slowly and listen to your body; build up exercise slowly and engage in activities you enjoy.

IMPORTANT: If you have not been exercising regularly or are still going through treatment, please consult with your physician before engaging in exercise. People who are going through radiation should avoid chlorine exposure because it may irritate the skin.

Survivors with severe anemia should delay activity until anemia improves. Survivors with compromised immune systems should avoid public gyms until their white blood cell counts return to normal.

Building Strength

It will probably come as no surprise to you that exercise can build strength, particularly exercises that continually challenge your muscles. This is well known, but what about mental strength? Can regular exercise do more than just increase the poundage we can lift?

In Ashley's story she mentioned the kayak trip she went on. This is a great example of the healing effect that physical activity and adventure can provide. On this expedition she was surrounded by women around her age who were coping with the same emotions, setbacks, and scars and they battled the river together. This is an example of building character and strength, both physical and mental. (For more information on expeditions, see the resources section at the end of this chapter.) There is just no feeling like accomplishing a task you never thought you would be able to, surrounded by people who are, without a doubt, with you every step of the way.

There is a power in achieving; there is a strength in stepping outside the boundaries of what you think is possible. Have you ever tried rock climbing? Kayaking? Snowboarding? I cannot encourage you enough to try something new (get a class, instructor, or someone experienced to go with you). Although the classic gym workouts definitely add physical strength and build strength of character, trying new activities on for size can increase this effect dramatically. There are many other reasons to add a variety of activities into your daily routine: enjoyment, cross-training, motivation, meeting new people, developing new skills, and the list goes on. Search online for opportunities in your area; you may be surprised of the organizations, facilities, and options available.

No one knows the physical, emotional, and spiritual healing power of adventure better than Mike Lang, who, after being diagnosed and treated for Hodgkin's lymphoma, started Survive & Thrive Expeditions. Survive & Thrive expeditions are adventure travel trips for young adult cancer survivors; this group is who Ashley went kayaking with. This is what Mike has to say when asked about exercise:

> On our expeditions most people say that they have never felt so good since finishing treatments. Some actually have phoned us afterwards to ask for the trip menu because they think it is the food on the trip that made them feel so great. But backcountry food is not actually very healthy, and I always tell them: "It's not the food! It's all the paddling, hiking, and swimming that made you feel so great!" Almost 100 percent of young adult cancer survivors that come on our trips are amazed at what their bodies can still do. All they need is the opportunity to rediscover their strength and vitality after months or years of being told what is wrong with their bodies. They need to have their eyes opened to the fact that there are still a billion things in their body working perfectly...and physical activity is the best way to show them that!

Not ready to try something completely new? What about hiking or walking in a new location close to home or away? It can also be used as a goal—something to train toward. As an example, I have "Climb Mount Kilimanjaro" on my life list (aka bucket list). I would need to train for such a hike, perhaps do some hill runs in the city or escape to some more local national parks to hike up into higher altitude.

Nutrition and Cancer

Although numerous studies link nutritional intake with an increased risk of certain types of cancer, it is important to remember that it is only an association and not necessarily a direct causative effect. There will always be people who eat poorly and never develop cancer, and there will inevitably be people who eat very healthily who do develop cancer. There are many factors at play in the development of cancers, but why not do our best to modify the lifestyle factors that may reduce risk of developing cancers and other chronic conditions? Many risk factors, such as genetics, are beyond our control, but we *do* usually have control over our physical activity and nutritional intake.

Nutrition and Cancer Prevention

Experts agree that proper nutrition can play an important role in reducing our risk for developing many types of cancer. A report by the World Cancer Research Fund/American Institute for Cancer Research (WCRF/AICR) presents a compilation of cancer research that shows there is probable or convincing evidence that the risk of developing certain cancers can increase or decrease based on the intake of many different types of food.[1]

Foods that were found to increase risk of developing certain cancers include:

- Alcoholic beverages (mouth, pharynx, larynx, esophageal, liver, colorectal, and breast)
- Red meat (colorectal)
- Processed meat (colorectal)
- Salt or salty foods (stomach)

Foods that were found to reduce risk of developing certain cancers include:

- Foods high in dietary fibre, such as fruit, vegetables, whole grains, beans, and lentils (colorectal)

- Non-starchy vegetables, such as green leafy vegetables (i.e., lettuce and spinach), broccoli, okra, eggplant, and bok choy (mouth, pharynx, larynx, esophageal, and stomach)
- Fruits (mouth, pharynx, larynx, esophageal, lung, and stomach)
- Garlic (colorectal)
- Fluid milk (colorectal)
- Foods containing folate such as fortified cereals and grains, lentils, beans, and spinach (pancreatic)
- Foods containing carotenoids, such as fish, eggs, pumpkin, winter squash, carrots, sweet potatoes, red peppers, and cantaloupe (mouth, pharynx, larynx, and lung)
- Foods containing lycopene, such as tomatoes and tomato products (prostate)
- Foods containing selenium, such as tuna, pork, poultry, Brazil nuts, and grain products (prostate)

As you can see, not all foods are associated with an increased or reduced risk of all types of cancer. This is likely because different forms of cancer can involve very different disease pathways. In general, incorporating foods from all food groups into a balanced diet will help to reduce your risk for cancer. The same WCRF/AICR report mentioned above also outlines a list of some specific recommendations to reduce your risk for developing cancer through dietary intake:

1. Achieving and maintaining a healthy body weight throughout life: This is likely one of the most important ways to protect against cancer, and it also helps to protect against the development of a number of chronic diseases, such as diabetes or heart disease.
2. Limit your intake of energy-dense, nutrient-poor foods (such as highly processed foods, fast food, and baked goods) to maximize intake of nutrient-rich foods and promote a healthy body weight.
3. Avoid sugar-sweetened beverages, which contribute significantly

to the North American daily calorie intake and contribute to the global rise in obesity rates.

4. Eat mostly foods of plant origin, such as fruits, vegetables, and whole grains.

5. Limit your intake to no more than 300 g or 11 oz of cooked red meat per week (about four *Food Guide* servings per week; note, however, that most restaurant portion sizes range from 8 to 12 oz for steak) and eat very little (if any) processed meat.

6. Limit or avoid alcohol: In terms of cancer risk, any alcohol consumption was found to increase risk for several types of cancer. If alcohol is consumed, limit intake to no more than two drinks per day for men and one drink per day for women. Evidence shows that the type of alcohol consumed does not matter when it comes to cancer risk; all intake may have potentially harmful effects.

7. Limit your intake of salt, which has a clear relationship with the development of stomach cancer. Most North Americans are eating double or triple the recommended amount of sodium every day! (The majority comes from processed, packaged, or convenience foods.)

8. Aim to meet your nutrient needs through diet alone, as evidence shows that supplements can sometimes do more harm than good. A few exceptions do exist, such as the recommendation of vitamin D supplementation for those with limited sunlight exposure, vitamin B12 for those who have been diagnosed with a limited ability to absorb this vitamin, or if a clinical nutrient deficiency has been detected by your doctor and cannot be managed through diet alone. A regular strength multivitamin may generally be taken without concern, although whether any true benefit is conferred is uncertain. Always use dietary supplements in consultation with a health professional such as your doctor, pharmacist, or a registered dietitian.

I am often asked about organic foods for cancer prevention or management. There is currently a lack of research to demonstrate whether organic foods or foods produced by other farming and production methods influence the incidence, progression, or recurrence of cancer.[4]

When You Have Cancer: Managing Side Effects

Many of the unfortunate side effects of medical cancer therapy impact our ability to eat normally. Each person's response to therapy is different, but common examples of side effects include changes in taste or smell, dry mouth, food cravings or aversions, heartburn, loss of appetite, increased appetite, swallowing difficulties, and gastrointestinal issues such as constipation, diarrhea, gas, bloating, or cramping. The Canadian Cancer Society publication *Eating Well When You Have Cancer* provides practical guidance and suggestions for dealing with these common side effects. Proper nutrition throughout treatment is important because the body's metabolism is often altered by the cancerous state.[7]

Food safety is an extremely important consideration during therapy in which the immune system is compromised; ensure that all meat, fish, eggs, and poultry are fully cooked and avoid cross-contamination. A common concern among many individuals diagnosed with cancer is sugar intake, as many believing that sugar "feeds" cancer cells. Research has shown that sugar intake does not directly increase the risk for progression of cancer; however, many foods and beverages that are high in added sugars are contributors to excess body weight and may displace foods of higher nutritional value.[4] Thus, as is recommended for the general population, limiting intake of foods or beverages high in added sugars is suggested.

Achieving and maintaining optimal nutritional status throughout the cancer process can be extremely difficult, and management of treatment side effects is crucial for maintaining adequate intake. Cancer treatment centres generally have one or more registered dietitians on staff to help clients to manage nutritional and weight issues throughout therapy.

Healthy Eating in Long Term Survivorship

Much nutrition research to date has been focused on cancer prevention, with those in long-term cancer survivorship long being left without much guidance of how to eat following the end of their treatment, although recent research in this area is beginning to expand. The present recommendations from the Canadian Cancer Society and the American Cancer Society suggest that this group of individuals should receive ongoing nutritional care from a trained professional, such as a registered dietitian, and that unless otherwise directed would benefit from following the recommendations listed above for nutrition and cancer prevention and by achieving and maintaining a healthy body weight through a balanced diet and regular physical activity. As noted above in the cancer prevention recommendations, the use of dietary supplements has also not been proven to reduce risk for recurrence or improve outcomes for cancer survivors (except in circumstances of demonstrated clinical nutrient deficiencies or when dietary intake of a nutrient is consistently low). Aim to meet nutrition requirements through food alone unless directed by a member of your medical team.

There is increasing evidence that being overweight or obese increases the risk of cancer recurrence and reduces overall survival among persons diagnosed with cancer.[4] Eating a diet that is rich in vegetables and fruit, incorporates balance and variety using the four food groups, and limits alcohol consumption may sound like a boring route to take. However, in this case it is difficult to argue against the great deal of evidence that has been found in the area of cancer research that shows the benefit of balanced nutrition. While weight stability is promoted during active cancer treatment, it is thought that medically supervised intentional weight loss of one to two lbs per week achieved through healthy eating practices and physical activity in overweight survivors following treatment may be beneficial.[4]

In survivors who are underweight and/or malnourished during or following treatment, further weight loss is not recommended and can lead to delays in treatment or healing, increase risk for complications, and reduce quality of life. In these circumstances, focus on increasing food intake from healthy sources to optimize nutrition and promote weight gain in consultation with the medical team.[4]

For more information about healthy eating, see Chapter 13: Eating for Life.

Resources

Wellspring: A lifetime of Cancer Support—*www.wellspring.ca*
Behavioural Medicine Laboratory, University of Alberta—*www.behaviouralmedlab.ualberta.ca*
Life into Days—*www.lifeintodays.com*
World Cancer Research Fund—Food, Nutrition, Physical Activity, and the Prevention of Cancer—*www.dietandcancerreport.org*
Survive and Thrive Expeditions—*www.survivethrive.org*

References

1. World Cancer Research Fund/American Institute for Cancer Research. Food, Nutrition, Physical Activity, and the Prevention of Cancer: a Global Perspective. Washington. DC: AICR, 2007. Available online at: www.dietandcancerreport.org.

2. Meyerhardt, JA et al. (2006). Impact of physical activity on cancer recurrence and survival in patients with stage III colon cancer: findings from CALGB 89803. *J Clin Oncol.*; 24(22): 3535-41.

3. Friedenreich, C & MR Orenstein. Physical activity and cancer prevention: Etiologic evidence and biological mechanisms. International Research Conference on Food, Nutrition & Cancer. Washington, DC: July 11-12, 2002 pp. 3456S-3464S.

4. Rock, CL et al. Nutrition and physical activity guidelines for cancer survivors. *CA Cancer J Clin.* 2012; 62: 242–74.

5. Courneya, KS et al. (2007). Effects of aerobic and resistance exercise in breast cancer patients receiving adjuvant chemotherapy: A multicenter randomized control trial. *Journal of Clinical Oncology*, 25(28), 4396-4404.

6. McNeely, ML & KS Courneya. (2010). Exercise programs for cancer-related fatigue: evidence and clinical guidelines. *J Natl Compr Canc Netw*, 8(8): 945-53.

7. Canadian Cancer Society. (2008). Eating Well When You Have Cancer. Available online at: www.cancer.ca.

Chapter 9

Multiple Sclerosis and Mobility: Overcoming Barriers

"Literally overnight my world completely changed. I went from worrying about my 500 m [speed skating] time to wondering if I could make it down the stairs."
— Crystal Phillips

Crystal Phillips was at the peak of a speed skating career when a crushing diagnosis of multiple sclerosis turned her world upside down. Eventually realizing that she truly knows her body best allowed Crystal to overcome many of the barriers that others had set for her based solely on her diagnosis. Her story is one of resilience, empowerment, and giving back. Following Crystal's story we will discuss information and recent research in the areas of physical activity and nutrition in multiple sclerosis.

Crystal's Story

There will always be many challenges that you need to face and overcome to make yourself stronger and to push yourself mentally and physically harder than you ever thought possible. In the spring of 2005, I faced one of my biggest challenges.

It started with a tingly foot one morning. The next day the tingly numb feeling progressed into both my legs up to my knees.

That night at about 4 am I could barely feel half my body, so my roommate drove me to the hospital. The following two days saw me through a battery of tests as the numbness quickly progressed up to my chest. On the third day of being at the hospital and waiting patiently for the MRI results with my mom by my side, a team of neurologists walked in with a look I'll never forget. My stomach started to turn as they said good morning with a nervous tone to their voices. They went into a lengthy explanation using words I did not understand until the end when they said: "This is also known as multiple sclerosis, or MS."

The first thing I thought was that I was going to be in a wheelchair in the matter of a couple weeks and eventually die from the disease. All my goals and dreams seemed to have been snatched away. After moments of silence and crying, the neurologists explained that the disease is not a death sentence. They tried to encourage me by telling me that I could lead a pretty normal life, but all I wanted to know was whether I could still skate. The doctor looked at me steadily and told me that any physical activity as strenuous as speed skating would only exacerbate the symptoms. It was in my best interest to never skate again.

Literally overnight my world completely changed. I went from worrying about my 500 m time to wondering if I could make it down the stairs. But I kept my goal in mind: to return to the ice.

It took me four long months to recover and get used to the daily injections I now had to take, but as soon as I could, I started training again. At first I eased my way back into training but was impatient and feeling so far behind my competition. I used anger and frustration to push myself harder and harder. Three months into the season I raced my first competition. The races were exceptionally exhausting, but I continued to skate all four distances (500 m, 1,000 m, 1,500 m, and 3,000 m) instead of listening to my body. All things considered, I skated well but was still nowhere near where I left off and it still felt like I was teaching a new body what to do. That weekend was not only physically exhausting, but because I put a lot of pressure on myself and had set unrealistic expectations, I was stressed out mentally as well.

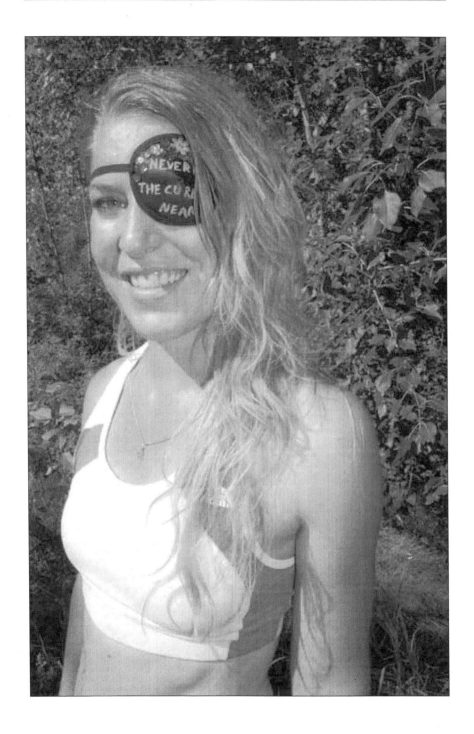

Two days after the competition, I woke up without any feeling on the entire left side of my body. That's when reality hit me: I have multiple sclerosis. I did not truly believe or accept what had happened in the spring. I needed that relapse to truly understand that I will have to deal with this lifelong illness with no cure.

This was my major turning point. I knew that something needed to change and I was tired of feeling sorry for myself. I decided to take my parents' tough love advice and turn my negative situation into a positive one. I also decided that I wanted to take more control over my health instead of leaving my future in my doctors' hands when I know my body best.

It's amazing where a simple mental shift, from negative thoughts to positive thoughts, can take you.

Starting from when I was about twelve years old, I rode with my sisters and friends in the MS Bike Tour from Leduc to Camrose. None of us really knew what MS was or knew anyone who had the disease, but we kept riding each year because it was fun. Remembering how fun this ride was, I decided to create a team of my own that year and hopefully get a few friends and family to ride with me. So I started to rally my family, friends, and supporters to join me in the Airdrie to Olds RONA MS Bike Tour in 2006. Before I knew it, I was captaining one of the largest teams in North America consisting of 88 members and raising a rookie team record of $56,000. I continued leading a team in the MS Bike Tour for four more years raising over $265,000 for MS research.

Over the years I also chose to be more proactive with my health. I started with speaking with doctors and neurologists, poring over medical books and studies, and researching what options I had. Again and again, I received the same advice: "You cannot be physically active with MS. You'll overheat, fatigue, and wear yourself out. It's too dangerous." But I knew that exercise in the right amounts made me feel better, not worse. So, once again, I eased myself back into my skating program. Most days I forgot I even had MS, but the odd day, my legs would start going numb—a red flag I learned to appreciate as a warning to slow down and rest.

Off the ice, I was discovering the power of good nutrition. I filled my diet with nutrient-dense foods, stocked my cupboard with good quality supplements, and slowly began to eliminate anything "artificial" in both my foods and cosmetics. The results were almost immediate, giving me more energy and confidence to take control of my health. My skating started to improve again and my symptoms lessened. I was so inspired that I enrolled in the Canadian School of Natural Nutrition. For two years I studied natural nutrition, graduating in 2008 as a Registered Holistic Nutritionist.

Despite feeling better and with continued daily self-injections, my annual MRI showed new/active damage in my brain and spinal column each year. A little discouraged, I once again started researching my options. Doctors told me a different drug, more powerful but with more side effects, would be a better treatment option. But all the drugs, injections, and checkups had not only worn me out, they scared me and were always a discouraging experience. Without results to show improvement, I thought there was little reason to continue with medication.

In April 2010, I lost vision in my left eye. It is called optic neuritis and is the most common symptom of MS. After five years of daily injections, potential liver damage from the drugs, disappointing MRI results showing progression, and lost vision in my left eye, I decided to go against everyone's advice and go off all drugs and treat my disease 100 percent naturally.

After my friend Tobey heard the news about my eye, she came over with three eye patches, glitter, glue, sequins, and feathers. That night, Tobey, my roomie and good friend Laura, and I "bedazzled" eye patches! After telling my mom about this the next morning, she gave me the idea to bedazzle hundreds of eye patches to raise awareness and funds for MS.

Thus spawned Crystal Patches and the beginning of a new

dream to one day start my own charity.

Through amazing support from friends and family yet again, I started the "Crystal Patches—Keeping an eye out for MS" fundraising campaign, which helped me raise $35,000. The funds were enough for me to go to India to get tested for a new controversial treatment called liberation therapy not yet available in Canada AND enough to send my friend who also suffers from MS to get tested in California.

I went to India with my parents; two good friends, Priscilla and Shannon; and another friend, Donna, and her husband. Donna was also getting tested to find out if she would be a good candidate for liberation treatment, which opens up your veins if blockages are found to restore proper blood flow.

All of my tests, including a venography, showed that I was not qualified for surgery. It's funny to think this way, but I was devastated to find out that my veins were fine. I wanted them to be blocked so I could fix them and potentially cure my MS. On a positive note, I at least had an answer and information that I could move forward with. It was a different story for Donna. They found over 50 percent blockages in both her right and left jugular veins. Hours after getting her veins opened up, the rest of us got to witness her take her first steps without assistance for the first time in ten years! It was a truly amazing experience.

Nine months later, after my decision to go off all drugs, it was time for my annual MRI. I knew I had never felt better since being diagnosed, but it's the results on the screen that would tell me whether I was right. When the neurologist told me that, for the first time in five years, there was no progression of the disease, I was overwhelmed with happiness. Finally, I knew that my decision to go drug-free was the right one.

This news sparked more inspiration for me. After years of fundraising for the MS Society by creating one of the largest private donation teams in North America in the process, I decided to create my own charity focusing on the same complementary and alternative medicine that had helped me with my MS. In November 2010, my friend Graham and I co-founded the Branch Out Neurological Foundation, a charity dedicated to raising funds towards support and awareness of all neurological disease. The first event, the Branch Out Bike Tour in Panorama, BC, was a resounding success attracting 135 registrants and raising over $50,000.

I have big dreams of expanding Branch Out Neurological Foundation, and we have already been able to fund research projects at the University of Calgary and University of Alberta.

Along with my work for Branch Out, I am still speed skating, working as a nutritionist for a sport performance training centre, getting more comfortable with public speaking, and studying herbal medicine.

I can't help but believe that things happen for a reason. I am so happy to have been dealt a challenge that, with the right mindset, turned into an opportunity to make a difference and to inspire others to always believe in themselves and have the strength to overcome all obstacles to reach whatever dreams they may have.

Cheers to a healthy future!
www.branchoutfoundation.com
@CrystalPatches
@BranchOutNF

Exercise and Multiple Sclerosis

Multiple sclerosis (MS) is an autoimmune disease that damages the insulating myelin sheath of the nervous system that allows signals to travel along the neural pathways. As a result, people with MS can have spastic movements, impaired balance, fatigue, muscle weakness, paralysis, sensory loss, or numbness.

A diagnosis with MS can be devastating. It has the ability to turn your life upside down. Crystal's story is a great example of the power that exercise and nutrition can have on the management of the disease. Research shows that exercise can combat fatigue, manage symptoms, and improve strength, flexibility, and endurance.[1]

Research is powerful but difficult to collect because MS expresses itself in a variety of ways, making every diagnosis unique. As such, exercise may fit into everyone's life a bit differently and for different reasons. Here are a couple of examples.

Vanessa Charlton, the captain of my high school hockey team, was diagnosed with MS during her undergraduate degree. She is now teaching at the high school we attended. When I spoke with her about her MS, this is what she had to say:

> I can only speak from my personal experience, but I will exercise vigorously for one hour, five times per week, and sometimes even a sixth time. There is a psychosocial connection between my MS symptoms and stress, eating, and sleep deprivation. I find that regular intense exercise will release my body of any and all frustrations from the day, it will cause me to "shut down" and sleep well for eight hours, and it keeps my healthy eating in check. My workouts are extremely high on my priority list. Other than teaching at KVHS, I am also an employee of GoodLife Fitness and I teach both BodyCombat and BodyPump. My neurologist was so supportive of my wanting to become an instructor because exercise and fitness is crucial to the long-term well-being of MS patients. I experience the benefits of it every day because I have been living for almost nine years now with Relapsing–Remitting MS and I am not disabled whatsoever. A positive attitude also plays a huge part in living well with MS.
>
> That all being said, if I am finding that I am having a busy week or that I am starting to feel a little tired over several days, I will find a sub for my class or I will not

workout that day. It is extremely important to listen to my body. If my body needs a break (physically, mentally, emotionally), I will listen. Sometimes I will take a 30-minute nap after school before my class and that will make a huge difference. I will even nap outside in my car before a class if I need to. Ignoring those feelings of fatigue can cause that sleep deprivation snowball to start rolling and I always try to avoid it.

I'm also still playing hockey a couple of times a week as a little added bonus to my workout regime. I don't play on the nights that our ice time begins at 10:30 pm on a Wednesday night though. Yikes!

Of course, by sharing this story, I am not suggesting that most people with MS take on as much activity as Vanessa. To be fair, many completely healthy, young people are not this active. It is about finding what is right for you, what fits into your life, and as Vanessa says, listen to your body!

I had met the contributor Ann MacDonald at the Nike Women's Marathon in San Francisco. When I approached her, she was thrilled to provide her story, and immediately added, "You need to talk to my neighbour Craig!" It was a while before Craig and I connected, but we finally were able to talk. We had an hour-long conversation that seemed like mere minutes. His enthusiasm was infectious. I left the conversation motivated; the rest of the day I could not get some of his words out of my head. I shared some of his quotes and parts of his story with a dozen people that day. I am thrilled to share some of this insight.

Craig Washka was an avid cyclist before he was diagnosed with MS. After his diagnosis his body started to gradually deteriorate, so did his spirit. Slowly, he was no longer able to ride his bike. Through a series of fortunate events, he was introduced to the "handcycle" or "crank." His reaction? "YES! My arms still work, so why can't my arms become my legs? Why can't I train?"

This represented an "aha" moment for Craig, making the impossible, possible again. When the progression of your disease encourages you to stop moving, you must keep moving or the disease will win. Encouraged by the incredible people around him, Craig started cranking. The crank was a catalyst for him to start a series of events to get him (in his words) "off his ass and get [his] heart rate up."

His goal was to ride in the MS 150, but he set out thinking that if he rode even one mile, it would be a success. Every day he is taking it one mile at a time. Craig rescued a dog, who runs alongside the crank cycle. His theory is that if your dog is fat, you aren't getting enough exercise. At the time I spoke with him, he had cranked over 16,500 km in total and over 7,000 km with his dog. I have no doubt that by the time this book is published it will be many, many more kilometres.

His advice to others living with MS is to keep moving and doing whatever you can—it helps. He said because of his cranking he has more energy, is able to get out and explore nature, and probably most importantly, "get back into society." He also claims nutrition is a large part of his treatment, which will be discussed next.

There is no such thing as a drug free of side effects. Nutrition and physical activity are "treatments" that we all can use to release endorphins and increase vitality and quality of life, and, most importantly, it is something that WE can control.

When people with MS are creating an exercise program, there are some special things to consider. As Crystal mentioned in her stories, her doctors warned her about overheating. This is a legitimate concern; however, exercising in cool environments can help reduce this risk. Examples include arenas, air-conditioned facilities, or keeping the temperature cool in the room where you are exercising. You could also consider going outside during the cooler part of day, either early morning or late evening.

Other considerations would be exercising close to a bathroom in case of urinary incontinence. Listen to your body, as MS symptoms can vary day to day. Do not push yourself if you are feeling fatigued or think exercise is making any of your symptoms worse.

The American College of Sports Medicine has recommended the following for people with MS:

Mode	Goals	Frequency, Duration, Intensity	Time to Goal
Aerobic (cycle, walk, swim)	Increase/maintain cardio fitness	Moderate (See Chapter 5) 3–5 days/week 30 min/session	4–6 months
Strength (weight machines, free weights, isokinetic, bands)	Increase strength, power, functional performance	2–3 days/week 1–2 sets 8–15 reps	4–6 months
Flexibility (stretching)	Increase/maintain range of motion and manage spasticity	Daily Hold 30–60 sec 2 reps	Ongoing

Source: Durstine, JL et al. (2009). *ACSM's Exercise Management for Persons with Chronic Diseases and Disabilities.* (3rd ed) Champaign, IL: Human Kinetics .

Nutrition and Multiple Sclerosis

Anyone with access to the internet will find there is a great deal of anecdotal support for specific diets in people living with MS, such as restrictions on certain food groups, high-dose vitamin supplementation, or even incorporating very specific food items into the diet as a way to improve symptoms and reduce relapse. However, it is important to be cautious about overly restricting generally healthy foods or supplementing with mega-doses of vitamins or minerals, as the research in these areas is lacking. One relatively popular diet known within the community is very low in fat and allows no animal fat, dairy, gluten, or legumes. However, researchers have yet to repeat the results from a single study conducted over thirty years ago that stated this diet could be beneficial for people newly diagnosed with MS. That is not to say that this diet might not help certain people with MS, but as noted above, this condition is unique to the individual diagnosed. There are several different forms of multiple sclerosis, so it is unlikely that any single diet or food or nutrient will be beneficial for *all* people with MS.

Research in the area of nutrition and multiple sclerosis supports a balanced high-fibre diet that is low in saturated fats with a focus on healthier unsaturated fats (such as those found in fatty fish, oils, seeds, and nuts).[2,3] You might notice this is similar to the diet recommended for the general population. Crystal mentions gradually cutting out artificial elements in her diet. Many highly processed foods contain artificial ingredients, so replacing processed foods with more natural whole foods will generally provide you with a better source of nutrients.

A diet high in dietary fibre is important for many reasons; as discussed throughout the book, fibre helps to manage bowel health, which in itself is related to improved immune function and prevention of illness and other chronic conditions such as colon cancer. People with MS in periods of relapse or progression who experience difficulty with (or are unable to participate in) regular physical activity might be particularly prone to constipation. Maintaining an intake of 25 to 38 g of fibre daily (depending on body weight; the average female needs at least 25 g and the average male about 38 g), along with plenty of fluids, can help to prevent and manage bowel health issues.

Those with limited mobility are also at increased risk for low bone density or osteoporosis (this is true for all persons of limited mobility or low activity, not only those with MS).[4] Weight-bearing physical activity (where your feet connect with the ground, such as walking) *as tolerable* in conjunction with a balanced diet does help in the maintenance of bone density. Ensuring adequate calcium and vitamin D intake is important in the prevention of low bone density. Good sources of calcium include dairy products such as milk and yogurt, milk alternatives such as fortified soy beverages, and canned salmon with edible soft bones. Vitamin D can be difficult to achieve from sunlight alone in certain parts of the world (including Canada and the northern United States). General guidelines for supplementation in the general population in these areas ranges from 600 to 4,000 IU daily. I generally suggest between 1,000 to 2,000 IU per day in those with normal or mildly deficient levels. Those at risk for high blood calcium should be cautious with vitamin D supplementation. Ask your doctor for a blood test to assess vitamin D status, and they will be able to provide an appropriate and personalized recommendation for supplementation. They will then repeat the test in a few months' time to ensure the dosage is appropriate. There is emerging evidence to suggest that low vitamin D status is associated with an increased risk for the development of MS and other autoimmune conditions, but research continues in this area to determine whether this is truly a cause-and-effect relationship and if vitamin D plays a direct role in the prevention or progression of MS.[5-8]

Another common issue encountered by people living with MS is urinary incontinence. Managing fluid intake so that smaller quantities are taken throughout the day (as opposed to large quantities only a few times per day) can help to manage this issue. Other suggestions for managing incontinence is to be cautious with caffeine and alcohol intake, both of which act as diuretics and may worsen symptoms.

If you are considering any dietary restriction, it is important to consult with a health professional such as your neurologist or a nutrition professional with experience in this area if possible. This way, if you are planning to restrict certain items in your diet on a trial basis, you can receive sound advice on how to ensure you still take in adequate nutrients and maintain a balanced intake. Those with any difficulty swallowing as a result of the progression of MS should consult with health professionals such as their doctor, a speech language pathologist, or a registered dietitian for a proper diagnosis and help with the management of swallowing difficulties.

Finally, before starting any nutritional supplement regimes, have your doctor test your levels of micronutrients such as iron, vitamin B12, vitamin C, vitamin D, zinc, and selenium. If your levels are normal, there is little evidence to suggest that high dosage supplementation of any micronutrient will improve outcomes for those with MS. The theory behind high-dose supplementation of certain vitamins (for example, antioxidant vitamins such as vitamin C, vitamin E, beta carotene, and selenium) is that because multiple sclerosis is an autoimmune condition, supplementing with "immune-enhancing" antioxidants might reduce the progression or risk of relapse. However, we should learn from research in other areas that proves that what seems reasonable might actually be dangerous. When researchers looked at whether high-dose beta carotene supplementation might improve outcomes for smokers (who have an increased requirement for antioxidants in part to help counteract the cellular damage caused by inhalation of toxic compounds), to their surprise they actually found that high-dose supplementation of this antioxidant *worsened* outcomes![9] The use of any high-dose supplement is inadvisable without the ongoing monitoring of a physician.

In addition to Crystal's incredible story, both Vanessa and Craig also attest to feeling better by incorporating healthy lifestyle choices. Proper nutrition in conjunction with physical activity as tolerated, proper sleep, and stress management should all be considered important components of daily living with MS.

References

1. Durstine, JL et al. (2009). *ACSM's Exercise Management for Persons with Chronic Diseases and Disabilities.* (3rd ed) Champaign, IL: Human Kinetics.

2. National Multiple Sclerosis Society. "Nutrition and Diet." Available online at: www.nationalmssociety.org/living-with-multiple-sclerosis/healthy-living/ nutirtion-and-diet/index.aspx.

3. Eat Right Ontario. "Nutrition and Multiple Sclerosis." Available online at: www.eatrightontario.ca/en/Articles/Men-s-health-issues/Nutrition-and-multiple-sclerosis.aspx.

4. National Multiple Sclerosis Society article "Osteoporosis." Available online at: www.nationalmssociety.org/living-with-multiple-sclerosis/healthy-living/ osteoporosis/index.aspx

5. Ebers, GC, AD Sadovnick, & R Veith. Vitamin D intake and incidence of multiple sclerosis. *Neurology.* 2004; 63:939.

6. Simpson, S et al. Latitude is significantly associated with the prevalence of multiple sclerosis: a meta-analysis. *J Neurol Neurosurg Psychiatry.* 2001 Oct; 82(10): 1132-41.

7. Mirzaei, F et al. Gestational Vitamin D and the Risk of Multiple Sclerosis in the Offspring. *Ann Neurol.* 2011 July; 70(1): 30-40.

8. Raghywanshi, A, SS Joshi, & S Christakos. Vitamin D and Multiple Sclerosis. *J Cell Biochem.* 2008 October 1; 105(2): 338-43.

9. Heinonen, OP & D Albanes. The effect of vitamin E and beta carotene on the incidence of lung cancer and other cancers in male smokers. *The New England Journal of Medicine.* 14 Apr 1994; 330(15): 1029-35.

Chapter 10

Stress Management:
How Sleep and Stress Affect Our Health

"One day I saw a picture of myself and I looked like my-self...but in a fat suit. I did not feel my health declining; it seemed like it happened all of a sudden. Something needed to be done." — Sheldon Clark

It seems that we are increasingly balancing more and more. Our hypothetical plates are becoming over full and our stress is increasing. Long work hours, busy schedules, tight deadlines, family responsibilities, and high stress all directly affect our ability to take care of ourselves. When our lives get busy, and we seem to be juggling so many balls, self-care is one of the first thing to drop for most people. Here is the thing: Without your health, you cannot do anything you are intending. Your health is what will make you more productive in the end and help you to live longer in order to truly experience the things you would like to do. We talk a lot in this book about physical activity and nutrition as behaviours you can modify and have control over that will influence your health. In this chapter we explore other behaviours, sleep and stress, that you have control over that will directly impact your health.

Sheldon's Story

I have always been interested in business, competition, and the fast-paced world of technology. These interests have given me the privilege of working for some of the most powerful and influential technology and consulting companies in the world. What I did not expect was the toll that the lifestyle encouraged by these companies can take on one's health. The culture that is created at these companies encourages long hours and very little work/life balance, all the while delivering inconsistent messages about health and self-care.

I was working for a large consulting company where my responsibilities involved going into other companies to make them more effective. I would go in and work with the company to design more effective systems, or make the appropriate changes to save money. This involved a lot of travel, dealing with executives, and making many tough choices.

The expectations involved to work for or with these companies are incredible to say the least. For example, I would travel two or more times a week. Travelling can be a stressful endeavor at the best of times, but the consulting firm saw it as a great opportunity for me to take calls. It was the norm for us to be on the phone, mute it to pass through the x-ray machine at the airport, and pick it up on the other side so as to not skip a beat.

Our phones were assumed to be on 24/7; the company's experts on certain projects could be in the UK, Germany, or China and so would all be in different time zones. We were expected to accommodate that by taking calls at 11 pm or 6 am or keeping our smart phones on throughout the night to receive, and respond to, messages as soon as possible.

Consultants are usually on other companies' "turf," so it is rare they have any kind of schedule at all. This becomes very apparent in their diets. Many consultants try to grab a breakfast and lunch on project but are expected to remain in groups that tend to work late into the evening. This behaviour breeds disaster because by the time many consultants arrive at their hotel they are exhausted and hungry. I would get back to the hotel and order room service. Typically, there are very few options for healthy food on room service menus, and, due to exhaustion and stress, I usually chose a hamburger and fries or another fatty, calorie-dense meal.

Many consulting jobs are extremely stressful. An example of a particularly stressful job that I had was while the global economic recession was at its worst; we went into the company to help them cut costs, which meant terminating many jobs. During this job I noticed it was particularly hard to sleep and eat, and I felt an extreme amount of stress. Adding to this stress was my $250,000 of student debt. After graduating from my MBA at 32 years old, I had planned to pay off my debt by 45. This was creating even more stress and job lock. Combined, these factors left me feeling trapped, hopeless, and frustrated. I had very little time to think of anything outside of work, and when I did, I became overwhelmed with all I was missing and it started to feel like I was living to work.

At the beginning of every job, the group would sit around and discuss the needs of the group members over the project. Even when I expressed the need for exercise—and was supported by the group—social norms and group obligations made it impossible to break away for any kind of activity. Fitness became a big problem. We would also often have group meals at restaurants or order in to the job site to continue working over lunch or dinner. The preference never seemed to be for the healthy options. I remember a low point was going out for "lunch," which consisted of an ice cream sandwich. We got to select the types of cookies and ice cream to create the delight. While delicious, I walked away feeling guilty for the constant abuse I was putting on my body.

In saying this, it is important to note that when you look around many of these companies, the majority of the staff appear to be relatively healthy and fit from a physical standpoint. There are not many obese people, and there are even some individuals who I would call lean. There is a definite association between professional success and maintaining your physical image. These high-earning positions in consulting also attract people who have Type A personalities and will do their best to maintain their appearance. Where their health can really suffer is lack of sleep.

A close colleague of mine had a heart attack at 35. His hospital bill was $70,000, though thankfully he only had to pay a $100 deductible through his company's health plan. After this event he really took a step back to revaluate his life and the stress he was putting into it. He did change his lifestyle for a while, but a year and a half later he was back doing the long hours and neglecting his health. He has a family to support, health insurance to maintain (which is almost impossible to get after a heart attack), and, of course, social pressure. Society rewards going to a prestigious business school, repaying your debt, and getting a dream job...it becomes very difficult to leave. For my colleague, the prestige and stability took precedence over his own health.

I am now on the outside, starting my own company, and can reflect back on being in this system. I watch good friends of mine go through the same thing that I did. A friend of mine who is in banking said it is part of the culture to go out with clients and excessively drink one or two nights a week. It isn't like you can go and drink water; there is a tremendous amount of social pressure. She is a trader, and not many other people in her company trade what she does, so she is expected to be at her desk during the time the markets are open. Recently she had blood work done outside of office hours. She received a call saying there were some abnormalities and that she needed to go to a specific lab to get follow-up tests, but because the lab is only open during trading hours she didn't go. When working in high-stress jobs, health seems to drop further and further down people's priority lists.

As for me, one day I saw a picture of myself and I looked like myself...but in a fat suit. I did not feel my health declining; it seemed like it happened all of a sudden. Something needed to be done. I decided to take action. I started writing down everything I was eating and what activities I was doing. I started running, practicing yoga, and using the elliptical. I don't always keep on track, but I try my best.

I am now starting my own business and have more control over my hours. Don't get me wrong, there is still stress, but I am able to break away to the gym, go for runs, and have more choice about where my meals come from. I am back down to a healthy weight and this will remain a constant. Now my health will always be my top priority.

Stress

"Stress is like spice—in the right proportion it enhances the flavor of a dish. Too little produces a bland, dull meal; too much may choke you." — Donald Tubesing

We need a certain amount of stress in our lives. When it comes to a deadline or exam, a degree of stress motivates us and pushes us to get things done. Certain things in our lives, such as marriage, a new job, or graduation are typically very positive life events, but they can be very stressful. They can produce a large change in our daily lives. Too much stress, either positive or negative, can be detrimental to our health.

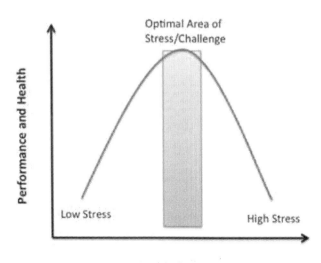

In ancient times stressors would have to do with survival—not enough food, threat to safety, etc. The concept behind the body's stress mechanism would be that we would need to fight off an attacker or run away (fight or fight response). In order to do this the sympathetic nervous system responds by causing our pupils to dilate, our heart rate to increase, our palms to get sweaty, and our blood vessels to constrict and increase our blood pressure, to name a few side effects.

In modern times the majority of stress that we experience has nothing to do with fighting or running but has changed to things such as project presentations, stock trading, exams, or financial burdens. The stress response has become maladaptive, especially when chronic.

Do You Have Excess Stress?

Too much stress can present in many different emotional, behavioural, and even physical symptoms. Symptoms of stress vary among individuals. Common physical symptoms include sleep disturbances, muscle tension, muscles aches, headache, digestive problems, or fatigue. Emotional and behavioural symptoms include nervousness, anxiety, changes in eating habits, loss of energy, mood changes, irritability, and depression.

People under stress are more likely to engage in unhealthy behaviours, such as using alcohol and drugs, smoking, and making unhealthy nutritional choices. They are also less likely to exercise than those who are less stressed. This is an endless loop, as unhealthy behaviours increase the number and severity of stress-related symptoms.

Here are some simple things you can do in your home or office to improve your everyday stress level.

Exercise is a very powerful stress reliever. Daily exercise can relieve overall stress and decrease anxiety and depression, but exercise can also relieve acute bursts of stress. A review of the studies on exercise and stress showed that people who exercise regularly exhibit fewer health problems when they encounter stress.[1] Try this: After an intense meeting, go for a short walk before returning to work. This will allow you to decrease your stress and to focus on the upcoming tasks.

Put *something that you really enjoy* in plain view in your home or office. This can be fresh flowers, photos, or something else that brings you joy. Try to change it or enhance it often so it does not fade into the background, and you always notice it.

De-clutter. Mess adds to confusion and feelings of loss of control. When feeling overwhelmed, cleaning up your home or workspace can be a positive first step. There has been research stating that at-work disorganization can increase stress levels; this is also true of daily lives. Sort and simplify.

Healthy eating fuels the body properly and increases energy. Although during stressful times we tend to gravitate towards sugary or salty unhealthy foods, this behaviour adds to anxiety by causing blood sugar highs and lows and decreasing productivity.

Eating regularly and healthily provides the body and mind with the energy and nutrients needed to fuel your everyday activities. As previously mentioned in Chapter 5, you should try to incorporate three or four of the food groups into meals and at least two food groups into your snacks to ensure that your overall diet is balanced in nutrients. To stay energized throughout your day, try to eat three balanced meals daily and add healthy snacks if your meals fall more than five hours apart. When you eat regularly, you prevent feeling too hungry, which usually results in reaching for foods that are high in sugar and/or fat and low in nutrient value. Stress can be exacerbated by hunger and poor food choices; taking time out once a week to plan healthy meals and snacks should be considered an important part of your routine to maximize productivity both at work and at home. Planning meals in advance allows you to take the guesswork out of what you're going to eat, which results in better choices, time savings, and cost savings. Taking time out to eat away from your workspace also provides a mental break to relax and de-stress, even if it is only for 15 or 20 minutes. The saying "You have to help yourself before you can help others" is important to keep in mind. Allow yourself the time to properly fuel your body, and you'll see and feel the benefits of eating well in both your work life and personal life.

Socialize and support. Spending time talking and sharing your life with people you enjoy being around can be a great stress relief and can create strong support networks, whether you are having a difficult day at work or are dealing with something more personal.

There are hundreds of studies demonstrating that having a strong support network helps ease the burden of stress, anxiety, and even depression.

Learning to say "no." It's well known that having too much on your plate can lead to excess and unnecessary stress. Most of us have many obligations to balance in life, such as work, parenting, school, volunteer work, household chores, social functions, and more. If you're feeling overwhelmed with your daily commitments, taking care of yourself by eating well, exercising, and engaging in other wellness activities is often the first thing to fall by the wayside. Admitting that you've got too much on your plate is the first step. Allowing yourself to be relieved of a few of your far-from-necessary commitments can provide you with some breathing room to take care of yourself. Don't be afraid to say "no" when asked to contribute your time and energy to something if you just don't feel you can give your best. Sometimes it's okay to be a quitter if it means that your overall stress level (and therefore your personal health and well-being) will improve.

This section was written as an ode to Lisa. Saying no is something that does not come naturally to some people. They want to take on the world and be superman/woman. However, having a list of priorities that separates the things that you can't compromise on from those that you can, can lead to reduced stress and increased overall happiness. As an example, one of my professors said that one of his "rules" is that family always comes first and he will never work on Saturdays.

The word *yoga* literally means union or merge. Not only does yoga promote flexibility and strength, it also promotes mental clarity and well-being through breathing and meditation. Please see Chapter 6 for more detailed information on yoga.

Massage therapy is recognized as one of the oldest methods of healing. Most people know that massage therapy can aid in relieving tired, aching muscles, which in turn promotes increased range of motion and circulation. However, massage also affects every other system in the human body. It has many positive benefits to our cellular structure in an indirect way. Massage stimulates the circulation and lymphatic systems to increase the rate the body will flush its toxins, and it also teaches the body how to relax. When the therapist is working on the tight muscles, it helps promote a "healing process" through a variety of techniques. Although the massage therapists do use their hands, other parts of their body, such as the forearms, elbows, or feet are used in the massage technique. All techniques are used to positively influence the overall health and well-being of the client.

Sleep is so important, not only for the regulation of stress levels, but for so many other reasons as well. In the next section, we will discuss the complex world of sleep and put some common myths to rest.

Sleep

It is not just consultants and investment bankers, people in North America are getting less and less sleep. (Add decreased sleep to moving less and not eating well...we really aren't doing so well.) The recommended amount of sleep is between seven to eight hours for adults and more for children, adolescents, and pregnant women. It is also important to sleep at the right time for you, which is when your core body temperature is at its lowest and melatonin is at its highest concentration. Melatonin is a hormone produced in the pineal gland that is part of your sleep-awake cycle. Essentially, if you had no reason to stay awake or get up in the morning, when would you be sleeping?

Sleep is when the growth and rejuvenation of the immune, nervous, skeletal, and muscular systems happen. Essentially sleep acts to charge your battery. Not convinced? Lack of sleep causes irritability, cognitive impairment, memory lapses or loss, impaired moral judgment, severe yawning, hallucinations, symptoms similar to attention deficit disorder, impaired immune system, increased risk of type 2 diabetes, increased heart rate variability, increased risk of heart disease, decreased reaction time, tremors, aches, growth suppression, risk of obesity, and decreased body temperature.

Many important physiological processes occur during sleep that are foundational to wellness. During a good night's sleep your body orchestrates the transition between different sleep stages to rejuvenate your health. The easiest way to demonstrate the importance of sleep is to look at the research when sleep is inadequate. Inadequate sleep has been associated with poor quality of life, increased pain, impaired cognitive function and performance, as well as increased risk of mental health disorders. It also plays an important role in your waistline. Undersleeping and oversleeping have been associated with increased weight gain.

— Dr. Mélanie DesChâtelets, Naturopathic Doctor in Vancouver and Burnaby, BC

There have also been links to undersleeping and overeating. A review of the research in this area was published by Cappuccio, FP et al. from the University of Warwick Medical School in the UK that included studies that represented over 600,000 participants from around the world.[2] The results indicated a consistent increased risk of obesity amongst short sleepers in children and adults.

We tend to take sleep for granted. If you have ever gone through times of sleep deprivation and then are able to experience uninterrupted quality sleep, you know that by the time you get your sleep, you feel like you are a whole new person. You are. You are working more efficiently.

Here are some things you can do to help improve your sleep length and quality. The list below is a mixture of sleep hygiene and clinical recommendations. For the clinical recommendations, I consulted with sleep expert and registered psychologist Sheila Garland working out of the University of Calgary.

Do Not Drink Water Before Bed

Drinking liquids right before bed can lead to disturbance in sleep caused by needing to run to the bathroom during the night. Try to stop drinking fluids after 8 pm in order to help minimize waking for bathroom needs.

Keep the Java (and Caffeinated Teas) for the AM

Caffeine is a stimulant that is consumed to keep us alert and functioning (and is a beautiful, beautiful thing). Keep your caffeine intake to the morning and switch to decaffeinated coffee in the afternoon, or avoid caffeinated beverages altogether.

Create Your "Schedule"

Getting on a schedule is one of the most important things you can do for correcting your sleep patterns. It will allow your body to keep your natural sleep cycle (circadian rhythm) on track. Try to wake up at the same time every day (even on the weekends). Your body will get used to the routine and, if you have gotten the right amount of uninterrupted sleep, you may be able to wake up without the aid of an alarm. If you are finding that you are unable to get up without the use of an alarm, or you find yourself hitting the snooze more than once, then it might be time to rethink the time you go to bed. Set an earlier time for bed that will allow your body enough time to sleep and recover.

Exposure to light is an important regulator of the circadian rhythm. Light exposure in the morning can help you "set" your biological clock and even make it easier to get your day started. You can do this by simply opening the blinds and letting natural light in, having a coffee or tea outside on the patio, or (my personal favourite) going on an early morning walk.

Get Your Body Moving

I like this one. We all know the effects of exercise on the body, such as decreased fat mass and increased muscle mass and energy. Aerobic exercise can also lead to better quality of sleep by alleviating stress and leaving our bodies relaxed. Some people (myself included) cannot exercise too close to the time they go to bed because it takes a few hours to get their bodies settled down. The ideal time for most people to exercise is around 3 pm. In the mid-afternoon, our core body temperature drops slightly; this is just when you start to feel a bit lethargic. Exercise gives you a boost to help you continue on with your day and have better quality sleep! Another quick tip is to do some light stretching or yoga before bed. This can calm you down from the activities of the day and help stretch out your muscles to prepare them for relaxation.

Business traveller extraordinaire, financial expert, speaker, and author Kelley Keehn had this to say about being active and healthy even in times of stress:

The more life demands from you, the more you must look at your health and well-being as an asset. If you owned a machine that had the potential to earn you at least a couple million dollars over a lifetime, you might look at caring for that machine differently. Your body is that machine.

The successful yet stressed business traveller has two options: They can listen to the plethora of reasons running through their head saying that they don't have the time or energy to work out and consume exceptional nutrition, or they can take control of their health and do what needs to be done. Taking the time to secure healthy food and be active simply has to be a must. Flights get delayed and sleep is often a much-needed luxury. But if you turn your business travel into an adventure worth exploring, almost any part of the journey can be more active, healthy, and fun.

No Nicotine

Do not smoke. There are SO many reasons why you shouldn't smoke, but for this section it is because nicotine is a stimulant and can disrupt your sleep. There are benefits of quitting smoking that are immediate and cause changes that you will see when you put down your last cigarette. For example, Health Canada's Tobacco Control Programme states that within eight hours of quitting smoking, the carbon monoxide level in your body drops to normal while the oxygen level in your blood increases to normal. Within 48 hours of your last cigarette, your chances of having a heart attack start to go down and your sense of smell and taste will begin to improve. Within 72 hours of that last puff, your bronchial tubes relax and make breathing easier, and your lung capacity increases. Within two weeks to three months of quitting, your blood circulation improves and your lung functioning increases up to 30 percent. Within six months, your coughing, stuffy nose, tiredness, and shortness of breath improve, and one year post-smoking, your risk of having a smoking-related heart attack is cut in half. Improved sleep is an immediate benefit that just keeps getting better with the increasing amount of time since your last cigarette.[3]

Only Intimate Moments and Sleep in Your Bed

The bed should only be used for sleeping and sex. Avoid doing work and discussing emotional serious topics in your bed. Try to avoid conversations—including on the phone—that provoke emotions while you are in bed. This can lead to added stress or anxiety when trying to fall asleep, which can make sleep next to impossible. You should also not stay in bed for extended periods of time if you cannot sleep. Sleep is not something you can "try really hard" to accomplish; the more you worry about it, the less likely it is to happen.

Sleep expert Sheila Garland states: "The worst thing you can do is to be worried about sleep. Worry usually leads to behaviours counterproductive to sleep, such as deciding 'I am going to go to bed early and try even harder to sleep.' Sleep is an important component to both mental and physical health, but it is crucial not to become focused on it."

Quiet the Mind

The longer you stay in bed, not being able to sleep, the more anxious and frustrated you are going to get, which will end up creating more problems sleeping in the end. If you are having a hard time getting to sleep, get out of bed, grab a good book, and sit in your favourite chair. Or do something boring such as folding clothes; think of tasks that are productive and yet repetitive and relaxing. During whatever activity you decide to do, try to avoid turning on any bright lights, as they can disrupt sleep patterns. For example, if you are going to read a book or fold laundry, turn on a small dim light instead of an overhead light.

You should establish a sleep time routine. For example: read a book for 30 minutes, brush and floss teeth, wash face, write in journal. Having some sort of routine will condition your mind to know that it is bedtime. We can train our mind to recognize a pattern of behaviours that indicate it is approaching sleep. The brain will begin to wind down and prepare for sleep.

Some of us will avoid negative intrusive thoughts during the day, only to have them build up and come to the surface when we do not have anything else distracting us while we are trying to go to sleep. One suggestion would be to take a half hour or so in the evening to problem solve and think through the day's events to hopefully avoid your ruminating at bedtime.

Disconnect from Being Connected

Extra light can interfere with our normal sleeping patterns. Looking at a TV, computer monitor, or even your smart phone stimulates the mind, making it harder to fall asleep. There are many research studies on this. More than anything, the waves emitted from any of these devices disturb your body's ability to fall into deep sleep or achieve rapid eye movement (REM) sleep. My suggestion is to move all devices away from your bed. If you do need to keep your cell phone on, keep it on the other side of the room. There was a time when I became used to having my cell phone on and within arm's reach when I was sleeping. I would literally wake up briefly through the night and check my emails and messages, sometimes even responding without a memory of doing so. This is extremely disruptive to sleep patterns and a maladaptive business behaviour.

Black Out

Introducing light into the room will stimulate the body into be-lieving that it is daytime and disrupt your cycle. Even early-morning light peeking in or bright city lights may disrupt your sleep. May I suggest blackout blinds? Those things are genius!

Write It and Forget It

Stress throughout the day can translate to bad dreams or inhibited sleep. Keep a notebook by the side of the bed so that if you do wake up because of something related to the stress of life—like a "to do" for the next day—you can write it down. By writing it and forgetting it, you will prevent your body from getting overstimulated and keeping you up longer than you need to be.

This is surprisingly how some of the greatest scientists have come to their discoveries. Otto Loewi won the Nobel Prize for medicine in 1936 for his work on the chemical transmission of nerve impulses. Years earlier Loewi had the idea that there might be a chemical transmission of the nervous impulse rather than an electrical one, which was the commonly held belief, but he was at a loss on how to prove it.

According to Loewi, he had a dream that woke him. He scribbled an idea down and he quickly fell back asleep. The next morning the script was not legible. But the next night the idea returned; it was an idea for an experiment to prove his hypothesis. He got up immediately and performed the experiment on a frog's heart.

This was the beginning. It took years for him to carry out a series of experiments that would eventually earn him a Nobel Prize and his title as the Father of Neuroscience.

Biographers have also said that Paul McCartney's song "Yesterday" came to him in a dream. He woke up with the melody in his head, went right to the piano, and started to capture the nocturnal tune.

These are just examples, and, of course, I am not saying that you will necessarily have a stroke of genius in your sleep, but it is interesting to note what our subconscious will do if we let it rest. Something about thinking while you sleep allows you to see problems in a different light. Also, these notes that we leave for ourselves can be very entertaining when read the next morning!

Feed the Need

Eat a small nutritious snack before bed to ease you into dreamland. The old wives' tale of cookies and milk had some validity. However, perhaps a healthier option would be better, such as toast and peanut butter, fruit and yogurt, cottage cheese, pita and hummus, or a small bowl of cereal or oatmeal.

No Napping...Well, Almost No Napping

Taking long naps during the day may prevent you from getting to sleep at night or staying asleep throughout the night. If you do need to nap, try to keep the nap to less than an hour—the classic cat nap—to avoid disturbing your sleep at night.

These are tips that might help you on your mission to get a better night's sleep. If you are unable to sleep or are still experiencing restless sleeping, make sure to follow up with your doctor to rule out any more serious health problems. I went through a bout of insomnia for three months; it is not pretty and it needs to be addressed immediately. Shockingly, coffee does not cure everything!

A good night's rest leaves you feeling invigorated and ready to face the challenges of the day ahead. It may also help you maintain a healthy weight and look younger and healthier. So try these tips and catch some z's.

Bonsoir!

References

1. Gerber, M & U Puhse. (2009). Do exercise and fitness protect against stress-induced health complaints? A review of literature. *Scandinavian Journal of Public Health*, 37: 801-819.

2. Cappuccio, FP et al. (2008). Meta-analysis of short sleep duration and obesity in children and adults. *Sleep*, 31(5) 619-626.

3. Health Canada. 2007. *On the Road to Quitting: Guide to Becoming a Non-Smoker*. Available online at: www.hc-sc.gc.ca/hc-ps/pubs/tobac-tabac/orq-svr/index-eng.php.

Chapter 11

Starting from Scratch
How Small Changes Can Add Up to Big Results

"The focus was on learning to eat in a way that would decrease my risk of cardiovascular disease, some cancers, as well as improve the quality of my life. Although weight loss was intentional, it was a side effect of these lifestyle changes rather than the main goal." — Ed House

It is common to put off what we need to do until tomorrow, saying things like "tomorrow I will start running" or "tomorrow I will start eating healthy," but as the saying goes, there is no time like the present. It does not matter how young or old you are and it is never too late to change habits: Ed House is living proof of that. Ed's journey is impressive, but it's extraordinary at his mature age. After his story we will explore how to change your eating for life and the first steps to getting off the couch.

Ed's Story

On my 73rd birthday I have the opportunity to share my story with you. I've made some incredible lifestyle changes and I now feel better than I have in years. Four months ago I was morbidly obese; walking up the stairs or putting on my socks were difficult tasks. It has not always been this way for me. As a child I was very active and worked very hard. I delivered papers every day and spent most of the day Saturday working on my newspaper route and playing sports. I enjoyed baseball, hockey, and especially football. Growing up, there was not much emphasis placed on nutritious eating. We did not have much money and ate the barest essentials of foods. The most important thing we had to worry about was finishing the food on our plate, no questions asked. This is a habit that is so ingrained and has stuck with me for most of my life.

In my mid-30s I experienced the loss of a child I loved dearly due to a kidney stone operation, I lived through a personal experience with cancer, and I underwent a divorce. These emotional, social, and environmental events catalyzed a trend of weight gain that described the next 30 years of my life.

I can clearly mark the day when things really switched for me with regards to my weight. An employment strike occurred and I was having trouble dealing with the situation. I was feeling down, stressed, and useless. At that time I believe that I started relying on food for comfort. This event was followed by a job change that involved more sitting and working with a difficult boss. I realize now that the way I chose to cope with the emotions of these events was self-destructive. I did not handle these situations as well as I needed to, but if there is one thing I'm very proud of, it is my drive to be a survivor. I've met numerous health complications. I'm both a cancer survivor and a stroke survivor. In those trying times I remember telling myself: "You have two choices: You can feel sorry for yourself or you can get up and do something." I always chose the latter. This was often a driving force in my attempts to regain my healthier weight. In fact, throughout my life I have made several successful attempts at losing much of the weight I had gained. It has been a journey. I followed very low calorie diets and with support I was successful at losing most of the weight. These results, however, were fairly short term and never sustainable. I felt good at the time, but these weight loss plans never addressed why I had gained the weight in the first place and the emphasis was on weight loss rather than eating to live and thrive.

At the age of 72 I hit a new low. I felt really awful—terrible actually. I was in a lot of pain and had very little energy to do the things I once loved. I knew most of my years were behind me, but I still had a strong desire to be alive and to do the things I love.

My lifestyle transformation journey began after a friend recommended that I see a naturopathic doctor. The focus was on learning to eat in a way that would decrease my risk of cardiovascular disease, some cancers, as well as improve the quality of my life. Although weight loss was intentional, it was a side effect of these lifestyle changes rather than the main goal. In the past I have had the tendency to give up and get discouraged. This program has been easier to adapt because the foods you eat make you feel good. I now know what healthy portions look like and I no longer overeat since I actually eat more regularly.

Five months later I've lost nearly fifty pounds and I still have a ways to go. In addition to the weight loss there was improvement of many of my ailments. I no longer experience heartburn and my bowel movements are better than ever. I am slimmer, I am stronger, and my cardiovascular fitness is better. My blood pressure has dropped and my laboratory results have greatly improved. I hope to decrease or even stop some of my medications in the near future— or at least that's what my family doctor told me. My motivation and energy is such that it now feels so natural to want to get up and do something. I have a new-found excitement and intensity about life. I get more enjoyment from everything I do. My exercise regimen started with walking and has progressed to include much longer walks and weightlifting. Lifting weights is something I enjoyed in the past and I'm so happy that I can do that again.

An unexpected bonus was the return of my erections. My family doctor had told me there was not much we could do about that at my age. Sex is one of the activities I miss the most. I hope with the cooperation of my wife that I can look forward to having sex again. If this isn't motivation for men to embark in lifestyle changes, then there must be something wrong with them.

Three months later my weight loss journey isn't over, but it is heading in the right direction. My quality of life has drastically improved. My wife and I re-engage in activities we had forgotten. I had hoped that I would feel this good and now I do. I cope with difficulties differently now and find much strength in prayer. I know most of my best years are in the rear-view mirror, but I can tell you that I feel pretty damn fine at my age—better than I have for years. If I had to say something to inspire others my age, I would say: never give up and don't underestimate the power of living a better lifestyle. If I can do it, so can you as long as you have a good partner to educate and support you, as well as a burning desire to feel alive. Every morning when I put on my socks, I think back to when I couldn't and that thought fuels me for the day.

Update: Since Ed first submitted his story, he has told us he can now run a mile without stopping, is off most of his medication, and has an excellent blood pressure of 110/70!

Lifelong Eating: Health versus Weight

I frequently meet clients like Ed who have spent years of their lives attempting to lose weight. The focus of one's life for a matter of weeks or months at a time becomes centred on the goal of weight loss, where every bite of favourite foods is "cheating" and one is meant to eat mostly cabbage soup or powdered shakes for days or even weeks on end. There are literally thousands of diet programs and products available in the marketplace; the US diet industry revenue reached nearly $61 billion in 2010[1] and Canadian spending is proportional with respect to population size, at an estimated $6 billion in annual revenue.[2]

The turning point for Ed, as he identifies it, was learning to eat for good health instead of eating (or not eating) to achieve weight loss. This wasn't about a number on the scale, but about finding a way of eating that would improve the quality and length of life. As with any lifestyle change, it is important to consider the long-term implications of dietary changes that we choose to make. The problem with dieting for weight loss is that it is thought of as a short-term solution to a long-term goal. The reality is, as soon as you resume your usual habits, you will be very likely to regain any lost weight because the "diet" was temporary. This can lead to weight cycling, in which you are repeatedly gaining and losing significant amounts of weight over a period of months or years.

Research has shown that the physical stress of weight cycling may be more harmful than being overweight to begin with,[3] with possible increased risks for cardiovascular dysfunction and gallbladder problems. It is thought that because weight cycling can lead to negative changes in body composition (reduced lean muscle mass and increased fat mass), health risks increase with multiple episodes of weight cycling. However, it is worth noting that these risks have been debated among health professionals and researchers for many years. Either way, the psychological anxiety and stress that the return of lost weight presents can lead to feelings of hopelessness, frustration, and depression, which may further exacerbate overeating or emotional eating and reinforce long-term weight control difficulties. (For more information on emotional eating, see Chapter 6.)

Although being overweight is associated with increased risk for chronic diseases, such as cardiovascular disease, various forms of cancer, and diabetes, it is important to note that not everyone who is overweight is guaranteed to develop these diseases. Many factors play a role, such as genetic predisposition for certain conditions, smoking and alcohol consumption habits, stress level, social supports, environmental factors, and other lifestyle influences; collectively there are many, many factors that determine a person's overall health status and risk for disease. In the absence of other factors (for example, chronic pain, anxiety/depression, elevated blood pressure, high cholesterol, or poor blood sugar control) it is possible that an overweight person can be a healthy overweight person. By the same token, we must remember that simply because a person is lean does not mean they are healthy. Thinness does not equal health. We need to consider the same factors mentioned above when evaluating overall health. Keeping this in mind, I guarantee that eating well and staying active will improve your quality of life regardless of your size.

Take some time to consider your long-term life goals, unrelated to body weight. Whether you hope to run a marathon, live to 100, see your grandchildren graduate, or travel the world, good health is an important prerequisite for most of our lifelong goals. In order to achieve long-term goals, long-term solutions must be sought. When it comes to changing the way you eat, think long-term. Ask yourself, "Am I eating a diet that I could maintain for the rest of my life?" If the answer is no, then it is likely too restrictive and not a reasonable long-term solution for your health.

Eating nutrient-rich foods most of the time is a great way to think about fueling your body. When purchasing food or drinks, ask yourself whether the item is nutrient-rich or simply calorie-rich. Nutrient-rich foods are those that contain plenty of vitamins and minerals and have undergone minimal processing; examples include fruit and vegetables, meat, beans, whole grains, and unsweetened milk or milk alternatives. Nutrient-poor foods are those that contain calories but little in the way of the vitamins and minerals our bodies need: examples of these include candy, chips, cookies and other baked goods, as well as highly processed or refined convenience foods.

For most of us, it is not logical to completely cut out a favourite food from our diet for the rest of our lives. Being overly restrictive simply leaves a psychological void that leads to craving that food even more. Following an 80-20 rule can help to keep your health in check while allowing for some wiggle room for treats once in a while. Once you have learned the principles of healthy eating, eat nutrient-dense foods at least 80 percent of the time to ensure that your body is receiving balanced nutrition and has the essential nutrients needed for optimal function. The remaining 20 percent allows you some room to eat the foods that are less nutrient-rich. This principle will also help you to consider your treats with more thought and consideration. Keeping a food journal can help you keep track of your habits and reflect upon your overall intake. Consider food as a fuel, and try new recipes with nutrient-dense foods in order to create variety and ensure you are still getting enjoyment out of food!

Read more about long-term dietary and lifestyle changes and tips for using food journaling as a tool for monitoring your eating habits in Chapter 13: Eating for Life.

Don't Sit Around Waiting for Your Life to Change (It Might Kill You!)

Have you ever really thought about how much time you spend every day just sitting? Whether it's in our cars, at our desks, on the couch, in waiting rooms, or at lectures or presentations, we usually spend a significant portion of our day just sitting. Some people working in an urban centre will drive one hour (or more) to their job where they will sit for eight hours (or more) and then spend another hour commuting back home. An expanding body of evidence shows that these types of sedentary behaviours that involve prolonged periods of sitting time are associated with a higher risk of obesity, diabetes, cardiovascular disease, certain cancers, and overall mortality.[3-6] The scariest part is that these risks still exist when planned physical activity is accounted for; in other words, going for your evening run or hitting the gym after work does not reverse the negative impact of sitting in front of your computer for the majority of the workday. These effects have been identified in studies addressing a variety of sedentary behaviours, such as watching television and other screen-based entertainment (computers, tablets, cell phones), time spent sitting in cars, as well as overall sitting time.[3-10] It has been estimated that adults spend *more than half of their waking hours in sedentary behaviours.*[11] In order to promote optimal well-being, it is important to not only eat well and be physically active but also to consider ways to reduce your sedentary behaviours throughout the day.[12] Start early with your kids: It is likely that limiting these behaviours in children and adolescents can reduce their risk of adult obesity.[13]

In order to reduce your sedentary behaviour, consider incorporating some of these activities:

• Walk whenever possible. Consider walking to your co-worker's office instead of calling them. Walk during your work breaks. Even simply walking around your office or house while you are talking on the phone can make a difference.

• Whenever you are sitting for long durations on a car or plane trip or in the office, make sure you get up and move around once every two hours. If you are on a road trip, stop and walk around or play Frisbee for 15 minutes. You may arrive a couple of minutes later, but you will have fewer aches and pains and will sleep better that night, and if you have a dog or kids, this is a great time to burn off some of their energy.

• If you just cannot give up your favourite show (which is completely understandable—there are some great shows out there!), place your treadmill or stationary bike in front of the TV. You can even take that half-hour you would have been sitting and doing nothing to get in a good, long stretch or do some rehabilitation exercises.

• Play. It is a concept we have forgotten about. Many people associate recreation or fun time with sitting behaviours like playing computer or video games, spectating a sports game, or watching TV. Why not join recreational sports teams or play tennis at your local recreation facility? On one of those really cold days you could play an indoor game of tag with your family.

• When waiting for an appointment or a plane, get up and move around while you wait.

It is time to get creative: How can you reduce your sitting time to less than two hours?

We all have to develop our own techniques to ensure we are not sitting for too long. For example, I have started doing 15-minute walks while I work. When I return I am more focused and productive. During late night writing, I have hopped on my exercise bike for short durations or even done something as silly as burpees or jumping jacks. If anyone was able to see into my condo window, I hope that they appreciated the entertainment!

Getting Off the Couch

Have you ever sat on the sofa eating chips, ice cream, or some other treat while watching a weight loss reality TV show and thinking, "Oh, I should get out and exercise…tomorrow" or "I will start eating healthy…tomorrow," and then continue to sit, eat, and watch?

STOP!

As mentioned in the above section, health does not have to be an all-or-nothing approach. You do not need the four-hour workouts they do on TV to see a positive change in your health. It takes 30 minutes of walking a day to see many positive health-related changes in your health; everything from your energy levels rising to lowering your risk of cardiovascular disease.

Ed's story makes a very important point: It is never, ever too late to make positive changes for your health. It is also never too early. There is no time like the present—but how? How do you develop a habit?

Think about your "bad habits." You are not actually addicted to the behaviour itself; you are addicted to the feeling you get when you perform the behaviour. For example, you are not hooked on sugary fatty foods. You may even regret eating a big McMeal, and wonder why you did. However, while you were eating the fatty sugary meal, your brain was releasing endorphins. We start craving and seeking out that pleasure feeling. When we repeat the behaviour over and over again, it becomes a habit. In brief, to create and maintain a habit, it must be enjoyable!

To develop positive health habits, you will need to find something that will create the same positive reinforcement. Essentially you need to trick your body into enjoying and eventually craving the positive health behaviour. Here are a couple of strategies to accomplish this.

Reward yourself. After you engage in the desired positive health behaviour, reward yourself with something you really enjoy or really want. Make sure your reward is not counterproductive, i.e., do not reward yourself with a milkshake after every time you run. Some suggestions of rewards could be a hot bath, guilt-free watching of sports, exercise clothing, or sports apparel.

Trick yourself. Like I mentioned, you have to disguise the health behaviours you may not innately enjoy into something that releases endorphins to aid you in developing the habit. For exercise it could be listening to music, enjoying new scenery, participating in a sport, or an accomplishment (climb a mountain, accomplish a "route" in indoor rock climbing, etc.). For nutrition it is a matter of finding the healthy food you love, trying new things, and adding "dip" to vegetables (adding something you enjoy to something you may not enjoy as much).

Make it part of your life. In order for a habit to stick, it must merge into your life. It should become a part of your life just as much as brushing your teeth. The best example I can think of is my parents' after-dinner walks. They take a half-hour walk every day after dinner. Their walks became such a regular thing that they would feel as if their day was off without it. I cannot tell you when this habit started, but I know it continues today. Even when they are travelling on the other side of the world, they still walk. I try to bike every morning on my stationary bike for 15 to 20 minutes to start my day off in the right frame of mind. It works well if there is a trigger to get you going. My parents' trigger is the completion of dinner; for me it is my alarm clock. For some people it is lunchtime or the coolest part of the day for their run. Think about what would work for you. A walk after work to de-stress? A yoga class at lunch? Or rock climbing with friends? To help develop habits, go through these seven steps.

1) Set a clear end result or goal

Have you ever hit the bull's eye on a dartboard when you were not looking at it? It is very difficult and next to impossible to hit a target you cannot see. The same principle is held true for health behaviours. You need to set out a clear target in front of you in order to work towards it. Although you may have a vague idea of what you like to accomplish (i.e., I would like to lose weight or I want to run faster), you need to work on your goals to make them specific, measurable, attainable, realistic, and timely (SMART, as you will see in Chapter 12).

2) Develop strong reasons to justify why you want the end result

Creating an emotional connection to your goal is extremely important and increases your chance of succeeding. Reasons could include being able to run a race in a certain time because you want to keep improving your abilities, or keeping active to be able to keep up with your children or be a good role model. The strong connection made to the reason for achieving the goal will help you overcome the obstacles in order to achieve.

In Ed's story you saw that he achieved greater results when he shifted his motivation from fat loss and appearances and instead took a health-driven approach. This is because he was able to make a stronger connection by focusing on living a longer, healthier life rather than fixating on what he looks like. This is very common. When the reasons behind goals are aesthetic, the behaviour can be short-lived when you do not begin to see results right away.

3) Educate yourself

Seems pretty simple: You need to find out what you need to do to accomplish the goal. For example, if your goal is to lose ten lbs, how much food should you be eating? How much weight is healthy to lose in a week? How much exercise, and what kind should you be doing? This information will help you develop a strategic plan to reach your ten lb weight loss goal. For information you do not know, I strongly suggest you talk with at least one health professional to help you make sure your information is accurate.

4) Prepare to be attacked

You will be entering a war zone, so develop a warrior attitude. Barriers to accomplishing your goal will be everywhere. Having a strong reason for wanting to reach your goal and a strategic plan will help get you through. The greatest attack will be internal; your mind will find every possible excuse to take the path of least resistance. Make sure you are prepared to fight back.

5) Get reinforcements

Changing a health behaviour needs support. Write down your goal and put it in a place you see daily; this will be a constant reminder of what you are working towards. It is also helpful to get support from the people around you (see Chapter 3). Let those around you know about your goals so that they can help out. They may even want to come along for the ride! You may also want to consider groups that have similar goals to add in behaviour-specific support. For example, if you are trying to run a half-marathon in a faster time, you could join a running group that will help push you to your desired speed.

6) Walk before you run

It can take 30 times of performing the behaviour before a habit can develop. This, of course, varies with each person and behaviour. It is this initial climb that is the most difficult. Keep fighting through this initial phase until these habits become part of your daily life.

7) Maintenance

Maintenance can be much easier than the climbing phase; however, it is normal to have small ebbs and flows in the behaviour. Do not let it bother you; lapses are normal. Life happens...don't be too hard on yourself. The goal is to not let the lapse last too long. Here are some tips to help get you back on track!

- Journal/Plan—When you can see what works for you, you can plan to make that happen. What time of day is best? What activity? With whom?
- Revisit your goals—As mentioned above, keep a constant reminder of WHY you are being active. Write down your goals and why they are important to you and keep them visible. Use visuals if possible—the finish line of a race, the picture of your child—something to bring emotional connection to why you keep working hard.
- Exercise with a buddy—If someone is counting on you to be there, chances are you will be. If you do not have a friend willing to do the exercise you want, join a class or group. You will be accountable to instructors of the class and other participants.
- Mornings—Set out your shoes and exercise clothes the night

before and get your exercise done right away. During the day you can come up with a thousand excuses not to go to the gym or for a run; if you get your exercise done right when you wake up, you do not even have time to make excuses and you will feel energized for the day ahead.

- Vacations or work travel—Choose accommodations within walking distance of places you want to visit. Choose hotels that have fitness facilities. Plan ahead on how you are going to get all your activity in.

- ENJOY!—If you don't like a certain machine or exercise...don't do it! Find an activity you enjoy and look forward to.

References

1. The U.S. Weight Loss & Diet Control Market report (11th edition). May 2011. Marketdata Enterprises Inc.

2. Mathieu, E. "Big Bucks, Few Controls in the Wild West of Weight Loss." *Toronto Star*. June 19, 2011. Available online at: www.healthzone.ca/health/diet-fitness/diet/article/1011436--big-bucks-few-controls-in-the-wild-west-of-weight-loss.

3. Brownell, KD & J Rodin. Medical, Metabolic, and Psychological Effects of Weight Cycling. *Arch Intern Med*. 1994; 154 (12): 1325-1330.

4. Hamilton, MT et al. Too little exercise and too much sitting: inactivity physiology and the need for new recommendations on sedentary behavior. *Curr Cardiovasc Risk Rep* 2008, 2: 292-298.

5. Katzmaryk, PT et al. Sitting time and mortality from all causes, cardiovascular disease, and cancer. *Med Sci Sports Exerc* 2009, 41: 998-1005.

6. Wijndaele, K et al. Sedentary behavior, physical activity and a continuous metabolic syndrome risk score in adults. *Eur J Clin Nutr* 2009, 63: 421-429.

7. Wijndaele, K et al. Television viewing time independently predicts all-cause and cardiovascular mortality: the EPIC Norfolk Study. *Int J Epidemiol* 2010.

8. Salmon J et al. The association between television viewing and overweight among Australian adults participating in varying levels of leisure-time physical activity. *Int J Obes Relat Metab Disord* 2000, 24: 600-606.

9. Hu, FB et al. Television watching and other sedentary behaviors in relation to risk of obesity and type 2 diabetes mellitus in women. *JAMA* 2003, 289: 1785-1791.

10. Ford, ES et al. Sedentary behavior, physical activity, and the metabolic syndrome among US adults. *Obes Res* 2005, 13: 608-614.

11. Frank, LD et al. Obesity relationships with community design, physical activity, and time spent in cars. *Am J Prev Med* 2004, 27: 87-96.

12. Hagströmer, M, P Oja, & M Sjöström. Physical activity and inactivity in an adult population assessed by accelerometry. *Med Sci Sports Exerc* 2007, 39: 1502-1508.

13. Boone, JE et al. Screen time and physical activity during adolescence: longitudinal effects on obesity in young adulthood. *International Journal of Behavioral Nutrition and Physical Activity* 2007, 4: 26.

Chapter 12

Goal Setting

We all usually have the best of intentions when it comes to our health and wellness. "I'm going to start eating better," "I'm going to start exercising again," or even more generally, "I'm going to get healthy." Often we have a goal in mind for our health, even if we do not label it as such. But without defining our goals, and planning how we will get there, the things we wish to achieve are all too often left on the back burner. Having no set goals and no plan to get there is like trying to hit a target you cannot see: impossible. Most of us wouldn't set out on a road trip without some idea of where we were headed. When we set out on road trips we use a variety of tools available to us, such as a road map, GPS device, or even good old-fashioned advice from those who have travelled the road before. In order to reach where we're going within a reasonable amount of time, we make a plan. Our life goals should be no different. This chapter will discuss the benefits of goal setting, how to set and achieve both short- and long-term goals, keeping track of your progress, and overcoming barriers.

Why Should I Set Goals?

Goal setting has many benefits. Whether personal or professional, goal setting provides you with:

- *Direction*—Setting a specific goal allows you to target a specific action or behaviour; it sends you in the right direction toward the exact place you want to go. There are many routes to wellness, so defining your own direction is the first step to success. Let your goals guide your behaviour.

- *Motivation*—When you have identified your goal by writing it down, it serves as an excellent tool to remind you of why your behavioural change is important to you. Keeping a list of previous goals you have reached is also a major motivational tool because it will serve as a reminder of your achievements.

- *Feedback*—When your short-term goals are time-sensitive, they allow you to frequently revisit the goal-setting process. Time-sensitive goals provide you with important feedback about how easy or difficult it was to achieve a specific goal, which tells you about your personal strengths and areas for improvement. Use this feedback to help you identify and overcome barriers when working towards your long-term goal.

- *Perspective*—All too often we get caught up with life's daily demands and forget to take time to think about what we would like to do or achieve for ourselves. Creating a Life List (also commonly referred to as a "bucket list") is a great way to bring perspective and balance into your life. Life should never be all work and no play. Have you always wanted to go cycling in Spain? Learn to cook in Italy? Go skydiving? Write a novel? Writing your Life List is fun, and checking items off your list is even better. For Life List ideas, take a look at Chapter 14.

Long-Term versus Short-Term Goal Setting

Two different, yet interconnected, types of goals are long-term goals and short-term goals. When many people think about goal setting, they think about things like losing 40 lbs, climbing Mount Everest, running a marathon, or being able to discontinue chronic disease medications. These are what should be considered long-term goals: They embody the end result of the effort you are willing to put in but do not provide you with specific targets of how to achieve them.

Short-term goals offer a step-by-step progressive way to achieve your long-term goals while making small accomplishments along the way. These short-term goals work in harmony with your long-term goals. The thought of achieving a long-term goal without having direction of how to reach it can be so overwhelming that it prevents us from ever moving forward toward that goal. We start thinking: "It is so far away. There is too much to do, so I will do nothing." It is often said that each journey begins with a single step. Identify one or two short-term goals as the first steps in your journey to long-term wellness. You can start working on your short-term goals TODAY.

Before setting short-term goals, take some time to consider what you really would like to achieve as a long-term end result. Write down your long-term goals to solidify them in your mind, and use them as motivation for your journey along the way. Think about *why* you want to achieve these goals. Using the example above, you can see that short-term goals allow you to begin the process of reaching your long-term goal in a manageable and specific way.

Example:

Let's say that you have a general life goal of eating healthier. You're starting from a point of eating take-out or convenience foods, snacks, or drinks three or four times per week.

Long-Term Goal: Eat a healthy diet to reduce my risk of developing illness and maximize my length and quality of life.

Short-Term Goal #1: Replace my afternoon snack with fruit or vegetables at least four days per week, starting today.

Short-Term Goal #2: Bring meals and snacks to work that were prepared at home in order to limit eating out or convenience meal/snack purchases to once per week.

Be SMART About Goal Setting

As mentioned above, our long-term goals, whether for general health or specific items on your Life List (as explored in Chapter 14), are generally quite broad in nature. They also often require us to be in a certain place in our lives that we have not yet reached. For example, for someone who does not regularly run long distances, it would be a daunting task (and truly inadvisable) to attempt a lifelong goal of running a marathon without some time, planning, hard work, and dedication to training for such an event. We all need to start somewhere, and it is up to you to decide how you want to reach your destination.

If your goal is health or activity related, it may help to visit a professional, someone who can give you an idea of what to expect on the road ahead and provide experienced guidance about the route. They can help you to determine the initial steps that are right for *you* on the journey ahead.

When setting your short-term goals, think SMART. This is an acronym that is commonly used to set goals for lifestyle change.

S   Specific

Your goal should target a specific behaviour to provide clear guidance for achievement. If your goal is too vague, it can be difficult to follow through. Since you are targeting some element of behaviour change, ensure that your goal focuses on a specific action or behaviour that you control and that can be changed.

M   Measurable

Establish concrete criteria for measuring progress toward the attainment of each goal you set. When you measure your progress, this can help you stay on track, reach your target dates, and experience the exhilaration of achievement that motivates you to keep pushing to your long-term goal.

To determine if your goal is measurable, ask yourself: How many? How far? How much? How will I know when I accomplished it?

A   Attainable

Ensure that the actions you will take to achieve your goal are realistic for you at this time based on your physical, social, and financial situation. Considering this during goal setting also allows you to identify and solve potential barriers to reaching your goal.

R   Relevant

Your short-term SMART goal should be relevant to achieving your long-term life goal. Ask yourself whether this is the right time for you to work on this particular goal. If not, there is likely another goal that you can set that is relevant for you at this time and also contributes toward your long-term goal.

T   Time-oriented

Since we are using short-term goals in order to eventually target and achieve a long-term goal, it is important to ensure that your goals are time-oriented. Similar to setting a deadline for project work, incorporating a time frame to achieve your SMART goal can serve as a powerful motivator and help you to continue moving forward toward your life goal.

Example of a SMART Goal: I will walk for 30 minutes, four days per week, immediately after dinner, starting this Sunday for two weeks.

For someone who has no significant physical limitations and is looking to become more active, the above example provides a

SMART first step toward increasing physical activity. It targets a *specific* behaviour (physical activity, specifically walking); is *measurable* by both the length of time to perform the behaviour and the number of days per week (which can be easily recorded on a calendar or day timer); has been deemed *attainable* for the goal-setter based on physical restrictions, time management, and social obligations; is *relevant* to a long-term goal of running a 5K race; and is *time-oriented,* as it specifies the total number of weeks that the behaviour will be performed in order for the goal-setter to review and set a new goal that further advances them toward the longer term goal in a few months' time.

Writing down your SMART goals and finding a way to track your progress (see Chapter 5) is an excellent process for self-discovery and change. A way to make your SMART goals even SMARTER involves:

E   Evaluate

Once you have achieved your goal and have consistently incorporated your behaviour change into your daily life, take some time to evaluate the process you undertook to reach your goal. Write some notes about what worked, and what didn't work, to create change. The evaluation piece can provide valuable feedback when you are considering your upcoming goals.

R   Reward

Rewarding positive behaviour change can help keep you motivated, and it provides significance to the fact that you've achieved something positive for yourself. Just be sure your reward doesn't come with the risk of returning back into previously unhealthy behaviours (for example, letting yourself smoke one cigarette after you achieve your goal of not smoking for six weeks). Rewards can come in many forms, such as a meal at your favourite restaurant, taking a personal day just for fun, or buying those shoes you've been eyeing all season.

Overcoming Barriers

Although changing your overall environment might feel like a daunting task to take on, consider taking the time to identify a list of barriers that are preventing you or those in your family or community from eating well and being active. Despite our best intentions and planning, it is inevitable that we will come across barriers to achieving our goals. Barriers can take many forms, and some examples include the following:

- Physical barriers (e.g., injury or illness)
- Social barriers (e.g., your best friend's birthday party is on the same afternoon as your usual cycling group ride)
- Time/scheduling barriers (e.g., your son has soccer practice during your only spare time in the evening)
- Psychological barriers (e.g., you feel too stressed out to cook for yourself)
- Support barriers (e.g., your spouse purchases sugary snacks that you have vowed to avoid)

It is unreasonable to expect that you won't encounter barriers to achieving your goals. Identifying barriers is the first step in overcoming them. If you are experiencing difficulty in reaching your goal, ask yourself why. If the barriers you identify are within your own control, what can you do to knock them down? If the barriers are out of your immediate control, is there something that you can do to change the situation for yourself?

Overcoming barriers is all about problem solving. Ask yourself a behavioural question such as, "How frequently do I purchase ready-to-eat or convenience foods?" You might answer, "Well, at least four or five days per week." (If you're not sure, take the *Convenience Food Challenge* found in Chapter 13.) Next, consider all of the reasons why you engage in this behaviour, jotting down your reasons on a piece of paper. Below is an example.

Why I buy convenience foods/why I haven't been making more meals from scratch:

- Not enough time! I work nine hours a day, and commute for two hours a day; work is taking up more than half of my day—11 of my 17 waking hours.
- All of my recipes take too long to cook and are complicated.
- By the time I get home from work and pick up the kids, I'm exhausted and starving!
- I never have the right ingredients to make the recipes my family likes anyway, and the closest grocery store is 20 minutes from home.
- I can't seem to get myself organized to cook much at home, and convenience meals are just so…convenient!
- I prefer the flavour of convenience foods to that of my own cooking.
- Fresh foods are too expensive.

Perhaps nutrition is not an area you are trying to work on at the moment. If you have instead decided to start working on scheduling in more physical activity, the same activity could be applied to this type of behaviour as well. For example, the number one barrier to engaging in regular exercise is reported as "lack of time." Here are some ideas to overcome this barrier:

- Schedule in exercise like a meeting, not to be interrupted. For fun, call them "Muscle Meetings."
- Wake up a half-hour earlier a couple days a week to get in a workout before the busy day starts.

- Conduct walking meetings with co-workers and friends.
- Walk around the field, rink, or court while you are watching your child or significant other play a sport.
- Plan active activities for family time, such as a bike ride, a game of tag, or geocaching.

Often, overcoming barriers will be about willpower and dedication to achieving your goal. The influence of social support is also very influential (as discussed in Ann's story in Chapter 3). Let your friends and family know that you have set a goal, and tell them why you're doing it. True supporters will help you along the way and will likely go out of their way to ensure that their actions or behaviours do not sabotage your efforts (although they may need a reminder or two along the way).

As you can see, we can come up with any number of barriers for any lifestyle behaviour. For this reason, it is only when we make something a true priority in our lives that we will be willing to come up with solutions to overcoming these barriers. Because we can come up with so many reasons *not* to change our habits, we must truly be motivated to change in order to follow through. It will always appear easier to continue with our current habits than to create change. Choosing even just a single behaviour that you want to change for the better may present multiple barriers; identifying these barriers and then developing a solution for each of them will take time and energy. Focus on your long-term goal to help keep you motivated during the time it takes to integrate change in your life. Knowing what you're up against allows you to use this knowledge to your advantage.

As mentioned previously, goal setting provides you with an effective tool for planning and achieving your life goals. The direction, motivation, feedback, and perspective offered by goal setting are invaluable in creating lasting change. Get started today—there's no time like the present to start living well.

Chapter 13

Eating for Life

"One should eat to live, not live to eat." — Moliere

Food has many roles within our lives. We eat when we're hungry, we eat for comfort, we eat to celebrate life's many holidays, birthdays, anniversaries, and milestones, and sometimes we eat simply for the sake of eating. Our bodies and brains are hard-wired to enjoy calorie-dense foods. From an evolutionary perspective, this design worked well in times when humans did not have consistent access to food and encouraged us to make choices that ensured our long-term survival. After all, there once was a time when we actively pursued our food in hunt and worked together to grow and harvest our own crops. How times have changed. For the most part, we no longer live based on these survival-type skills of hunting/growing our own food. In fact, we now spend relatively little time preparing meals that will nourish our loved ones and strongly influence a lifetime of health and well-being.

Most of us are well aware that what we eat influences our body weight, but we seem to forget how strongly this influences many other factors, such as our energy levels, emotional well-being, digestive health, immunity to infectious and chronic disease, and life expectancy. We all face unique barriers to eating well, such as limited time, finances, cooking skills, taste preferences, social pressures, and many more. However, with a little planning, I believe that any barrier to wellness can be overcome. As a society it seems that we have real difficulty in overcoming the short-term barriers to long-term health. We are a society of "here and now," and we focus on the immediate present instead of considering long-term consequences. Identifying barriers and goal setting can help anyone to start improving their wellness immediately. This chapter will discuss concepts for *lifelong* eating: You won't find suggestions for fad diets, radical restrictions, or detoxifying cleanses. What you will find is evidence-based sound advice for eating well to nourish yourself and your loved ones and some tips and suggestions for overcoming barriers to good nutrition.

Diet versus Dieting

For the purposes of this chapter, let us distinguish between the terms *diet* and *dieting*. When I use the term *diet*, the intent is to discuss the sum of all foods and beverages that we consume. We all consume a certain diet, which varies by culture. This is not to be confused with *dieting*. As a society, we often talk about dieting or "going on a diet," which implies that we will restrict something (or many things) we usually eat or drink (i.e., calories, carbohydrates, "junk" food, alcohol) generally with a goal of weight loss. The problem I have with dieting is that it is usually thought of as a short-term solution to a long-term goal. Most dieting programs are not intended to last forever—usually only weeks or months. The reality is, as soon as you resume your usual habits, you will be very likely to regain any lost weight because the dieting was temporary. In order to achieve a long-term goal, such as weight loss, a long-term solution *must* be part of the plan.

Many weight-loss plans have multiple phases or stages that you progress through, and they usually involve severe restrictions of entire nutrient groups and/or food groups in the initial stages before reincorporate them. These plans can be enticing because of the initially fast rate of weight loss (due to severely restricting some element of the diet, such as carbohydrates). As I mentioned above, we are a society who loves instant gratification. We fail to see beyond the short term for our long-term problems, especially when it comes to weight management. Many diet plans will tell you that most people who buy their products lose weight, but what they fail to tell you (and what they often do not follow-up with at all) is the long-term success rate of maintaining that weight loss in the following months or years. Research shows that in the long run, most people will regain the weight lost once they stop dieting.[1] For long-term health, consider your overall diet as much more important than any short-term diet.

Tips for Healthy Eating

"Don't eat anything your great-grandmother wouldn't rec-ognize as food." — Michael Pollan

Build a Balanced Plate

Using an easy 25-25-50 ratio and building what dietitians call a "balanced plate" is a quick and simple tool for controlling portion sizes and incorporating balance and variety in your meals. Start by including a source of lean protein (e.g., meat, poultry, fish, tofu, eggs, or legumes...any will do!), which will make up the first 25 percent of your plate. Next, incorporate a grain or starch product for the second 25 percent of your plate (e.g., whole grain pasta, baked potato, quinoa, or long-grain rice). Finally, fill 50 percent of your plate with fruit and/or vegetables (feel free to use more than one type of fruit/veggie at each meal).

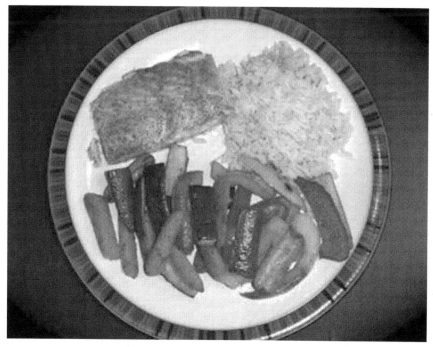

Photo: example of a balanced plate (salmon 3 oz, whole grain rice ¾ cup, grilled vegetables 1 cup)

Include Protein

Including a source of protein with your meals slows the rate of digestion, which helps keep you feeling full for longer. Incorporate a serving of lean protein such as skinless chicken/turkey, beans, lentils, lean beef, bison, tofu, eggs, or natural peanut butter with each meal to ensure that you are getting valuable building blocks for building or maintaining muscle mass, as well as many essential vitamins and minerals required by the body. Portion sizes for protein sources are ideally 3 oz of cooked meat, poultry, or fish; ¾ of a cup of cooked beans/lentils; 2 eggs; or 2 tablespoons of nut butter.

Fabulous Fibre

Vegetables and fruit are delicious sources of vitamins, minerals, and antioxidants, and also are the best natural source of fibre. Fibre helps maintain the health of our digestive tracts. Digestive health is actually a very important component in our body's ability to fight disease; did you know that the majority of our immune system lies within the digestive tract? Maintaining digestive health is crucial to our overall well-being. Help maintain your digestive health by consuming plenty of fibre-rich fruits and vegetables and two to three litres of fluid every day (fibre and water work together to bulk stool and promote regularity). Other nutrient-dense sources of fibre include minimally processed whole grains and legumes, such as beans and lentils.

Eat Regularly

I frequently remind clients that trying to start your day without breakfast is akin to trying to drive your car on empty. You end up with less than optimal results (and stranded on the side of the highway). Remember that food is not simply something we need to stop hunger, but the fuel our bodies need to perform their daily activities. Eating regular meals and one to three healthy snacks helps ensure that our bodies are refuelled for optimal performance throughout the day. Regular eating also prevents the feeling that we are starving our bodies, which can be helpful if you tend to overeat when your meals are more than four or five hours apart.

Our choices at each meal and snack dictate how we will feel both physically and emotionally for the next few hours. Aim to include three to four of the food groups with each meal and at least two food groups with each snack to have a balanced intake.

DIY

The do-it-yourself method is the gold standard when it comes to nutrition. Eating home-cooked food from scratch is ideal because it provides you with the most control over what you are feeding yourself and your loved ones. However, cooking a meal from scratch three times per day is not always practical. Try a few shortcuts to the DIY method that help save time while eating healthy: i) Batch cooking: cooking larger quantities of food and portioning into freezer-safe packages for later use is a great way to make the most of your cooking time; ii) Use leftovers: eating leftovers for meals stretches your time and your dollar while reducing waste; iii) Community cooking: start or join a community kitchen where a group of people get together and each person cooks a different meal; a few hours of your time provides you with many different types of meals to take home (and, as a bonus, adds variety and promotes your family trying new foods and recipes).

Food Journaling

Whether you call it a food journal or a food diary, tracking what you eat and drink on paper (or using an electronic application) can be a useful tool. This tool helps you to see not only what your daily intake consists of, but when recorded properly, it also allows you to track the quantity of food eaten, your eating schedule, how frequently you eat away from home, and, over time, allows you to make associations between food and emotions, energy levels, and productivity.

To complete a food journal, the more detail the better. Write down the day of the week, the time of day, everything you eat and drink including quantities, and any other notes you would like to incorporate (e.g., emotions before/during/after eating, location of the meal/snack, and how you're feeling physically).

Food journaling can be particularly helpful as a comparative tool if you have a goal in mind. For example, if you set a goal to eat seven servings from the vegetables and fruit food group every day, use the journal to count up the average number of servings you ate each day for at least three consecutive days. Compare your actual intake with your goal. Once you've consistently reached this goal (i.e., it has become a habit), try setting a new goal. For more on goal setting, see Chapter 12.

For the link to a detailed food diary template, see the *Resources* section at the end of this chapter.

Know What You're Eating

As you've gathered by now, I believe that weight stability is not quite as simple as "energy in = energy out" where the number of calories taken in needs to equal the number of calories you burn every day, nor that weight loss is as simple as "energy in < energy out." In fact, many clients that I see make the mistake of actually eating too *little*. Very low calorie diets (less than 1,000 calories per day) can actually cause your metabolism to say, "Whoa! Let's slow down or we won't have enough energy to survive." And a lower metabolism means fewer calories per hour are used at rest; you may be eating less, but you're spending less. The result is often frustration, in part because you're hungry all the time from an overly restrictive diet, and in part because the scale still isn't moving. Although you might think that skipping an entire meal (commonly, breakfast) would mean you end up eating fewer calories over the course of the day, research actually shows that those who report eating breakfast have a better diet quality, lower daily calorie intake, and lower body weight compared with those who skip breakfast.[2-5]

It may sound surprising, but I would argue that most people simply do not realize exactly what they're eating most of the time. You might say, for example, "Sure, I do. I'm eating chicken noodle soup." But does that soup consist of what you think it does? When you do choose packaged or convenience foods, be an informed consumer. The most important piece of writing on any food package is not whether it is "high in fibre," "reduced in sodium," or "low in fat." The most important piece of writing on any package is the *ingredients list*. After reading the ingredients list, you might realize that your chicken soup, which you previously assumed to contain chicken broth, cooked chicken, noodles, and spices (and maybe a few vegetables if you're lucky) actually contains about 20 ingredients, 5 or more of which you can't pronounce (usually stabilizers, food preservatives, and flavour enhancers). The beauty is, something like chicken soup is actually relatively easy to prepare yourself!

Take the Convenience Food Challenge: Open your pantry and refrigerator, or, for an even better overview of your habits, collect all of the receipts from all food and beverages you purchase for one week. Then make a vertical line down the centre of a piece of paper. On one side make a tick mark for every item that you purchased that would be used as an individual ingredient for a recipe to make meals or snacks, or was a natural whole food such as fruit. On the other side of the paper, make a tick mark for every packaged/processed item you purchased that was ready-to-eat or simply needed to be unwrapped or heated to consume. This will give you an idea of the proportion of convenience food that you're purchasing compared with food you're preparing on your own; many people are shocked to realize that over half (or nearly all!) of the food they purchase is purely for convenience's sake.

This problem is even bigger if you have very little food in your fridge or cupboards and you are picking up food on the run. Remember that the number one goal of any food manufacturer is to sell their product. Unfortunately, most of the time this means that packaged and convenience foods are laden with fat, sugar, and salt. This challenge exercise is useful for identifying areas for change. You might recognize that you only purchase ready-made snacks (such as chips, granola bars, "100-Calorie Snack Packs," or fruit snacks). Setting a goal to buy only unprocessed foods that make easy on-the-go snacks (such as apples, bananas, carrot sticks, or yogurt) is a great first step in the right direction toward regaining control over your diet.

Balance and Variety

It is not a stretch to state that in the typical North American diet, both balance and variety are often lacking. Balance refers to the quantity of different types of foods that are eaten, while variety refers to the number of different types of foods eaten. These are both important considerations for our overall health because they help ensure that we are getting the essential nutrients that allow our bodies to function optimally. Even the most active people can suffer from sub-optimal health if their diets are nutrient deficient.

The rationale for consuming foods from all four food groups (vegetables and fruit, grain products, milk and alternatives, meat and alternatives) is that each food group brings a different set of nutrients to our bodies. The table below shows just a few examples of key nutrients found in each food group; note that no single food group contains all essential nutrients for well-being. While some nutrients are found in many food groups, the quantities and specific foods in which they are found differs. Therefore, eating a *variety* of foods from each of the food groups provides the most well-rounded overall intake of nutrients to optimize our health. Buying in season helps promote variety throughout the year and provides the highest levels of nutrients found in fresh foods.

Vegetables and Fruit	Grain Products	Milk and Alternatives	Meat and Alternatives
Calcium		Calcium	
	Chromium		Chromium
Copper			Copper
Fibre	Fibre		Fibre*
Folate	Folate		Folate*
Iron	Iron		Iron
Magnesium	Magnesium		Magnesium
		Protein	Protein
	Phosphorous	Phosphorous	Phosphorous
Potassium			
	Selenium		Selenium
Vitamin A			
			Vitamin B12
Vitamin C			
		Vitamin D (fortified)	Vitamin D
Vitamin E			Vitamin E*
		Zinc	Zinc

*Certain meat alternatives such as beans, lentils, nuts, and seeds contain fibre, folate, and vitamin E.

Supplements: Friend or Foe?

As you have read above, variety is important for ensuring the overall adequacy in the diet for optimal nutrition. You may wonder, "Why not simply take a multivitamin to cover my bases and eat whatever I want?"

The supplement industry as a whole is particularly bothersome to me; anyone walking in off the street can easily and unintentionally obtain dietary supplements that may at best be unhelpful and at worst contain potentially dangerous levels of vitamins and minerals. "Natural" supplements can also be potentially harmful or interact with other medications you take, and are only regulated in Canada if they have one of three of the following: i) a Drug Inspection Number (DIN), ii) a Natural Health Product (NHP) number, or iii) a Homeopathic Medicine Number (HMN) listed on the packaging. The presence of this number is important, as it ensures that the product has undergone review by Health Canada for its formulation, effectiveness, and labelling and instructions for use, and it allows the government to track products for recalls, safety inspections, and quality monitoring.[6,7] Without advanced knowledge of recommended nutrient values across the lifespan, it can be a very difficult task for consumers to distinguish the good from the bad when it comes to supplementation.

Nutrition research has shown that there is a certain effect that occurs when we get our vitamins and minerals from food…an effect that is not replicated when the same nutrients are taken in pill form. The natural combination of nutrients present in food is best absorbed and used by our bodies. A number of scientific studies have shown that people who take daily multivitamins have no significant health advantages compared with those who don't supplement, although this is a difficult area to study since people are so varied in their habits and intake.[8,9] Further complicating the situation is that people who regularly take multivitamins or other supplements are usually more health-conscious to begin with, so it is difficult to separate the synergistic effects of healthy diet and lifestyle from the effects of supplements on their own. For healthy individuals who are consuming a well-balanced diet that includes a variety of foods, supplements may not be necessary (and can be costly). There are exceptions to every rule, however. For example, there are individuals who have known nutrient deficiencies that cannot be corrected through diet alone. Two supplements in particular might benefit many Canadian adults: a brief discussion of vitamin D and omega-3 fatty acids may help you decide whether either might benefit you or a loved one. Before taking any supplement, consult with a medical professional such as your family doctor, pharmacist, or registered dietitian to determine your individual needs and ensure it will not interact with any other medication you may be taking.

Vitamin D

Vitamin D is well-known for its role in the prevention of bone-related problems, such as rickets and osteoporosis. However, a growing body of evidence suggests that an optimal vitamin D status is also important in the prevention of many chronic conditions, such as cancer, diabetes, hypertension, and multiple sclerosis. Due to our northern climate, many Canadians do not achieve optimal vitamin D status throughout the year. Our bodies naturally make vitamin D when our skin is exposed to sunlight's UV rays, so our climate leaves many in our population with vitamin D insufficiency for several months each year.

The Canadian guidelines for vitamin D intake have recently been updated.[10] This is one vitamin whose recommended intake can be difficult to achieve through diet alone. The current recommended dietary allowance (RDA) for adults up to age 70 is 600 IU of vitamin D3 daily, and adults over 70 should get 800 IU daily. (All adults are cautioned not to exceed 4,000 IU daily from all diet and supplement sources unless medically supervised.) If you're wondering about your body's level of vitamin D, ask your doctor for blood work to test your vitamin D status. This will provide a better indication of whether or not you need to supplement and will allow your doctor to prescribe an optimal dosage for supplementation. Based on my practical experience, supplementing with 1,000 to 2,000 IU daily helps the majority of my clients to maintain optimal levels of vitamin D. If you spend much time in peak sunlight hours throughout the spring and summer, or if you're headed south to a tropical destination, you can probably skip your vitamin D supplement on those days.

Omega-3 Fatty Acids

Omega-3 fatty acids are long-chain polyunsaturated essential fatty acids, which are often lacking in the North American diet. Because our intake of these fatty acids is generally low, it may be beneficial for some to supplement with omega-3 fatty acid capsules. It is important to note, however, that all omega-3s are not created equal. Research shows that the most beneficial forms of omega-3 fatty acids are eicosapentaenoic acid (EPA) and docosahexaenoic acid (DHA). Extensive research shows benefits for neurological/retinal development, and ongoing research shows likely benefits for cardiovascular function, inflammation, and possibly mood.

Omega-3s have gained huge popularity in recent years, as research shows that many North Americans may benefit from supplementation (e.g., those at increased risk for cardiovascular disease). If you consume certain varieties of fish (cold water fatty fish, such as salmon, herring, or mackerel) twice weekly, you likely don't need to supplement on top of this. However, the majority of Canadians are not meeting these recommendations and some may benefit from additional supplementation. The decision to begin on omega-3 supplements warrants a discussion with your doctor or pharmacist, as these pills have the potential to interact with other medications you might be taking (such as warfarin or daily-dose Aspirin). If you're supplementing with omega-3 capsules, spend wisely and avoid the 3-6-9 combination; we already get enough omega-6 and -9 in our diets. Ideally, you'll be getting 1,000 mg of EPA and DHA in your daily dose (one to three pills depending on potency). If you have difficulty stomaching the capsules (a frequent complaint is "fish burps"), take this supplement with food or at bedtime, or try storing the bottle in the freezer.

As a final note on supplementation, remember that just because a multivitamin or supplement can be purchased without a prescription, it doesn't mean that it's not potentially harmful. I have seen vitamins and supplements on the shelf that contain levels beyond the upper tolerable limit of safety for any age or gender, so it is important to be informed about what you're taking and the dosage that's right for you. Try to get your nutrients from food first and foremost. Always inform your doctor and pharmacist about all vitamins, supplements, and herbal products that you are taking so that you can discuss with a registered dietitian whether or not you may benefit from supplementation while you review your usual diet.

Deciphering the Label: A Look at Food Marketing

"If you're concerned about your health, you should probably avoid products that make health claims. Why? Because a health claim on a food product is a strong indication it's not really food, and food is what you want to eat."
— Michael Pollan

I believe that a major part of the North American obesity epidemic relates directly to the food industry and the marketing of foods. We deserve honest information about the products we purchase, particularly those we consume that have a significant effect on our health. Unfortunately, the North American food industry has developed a nasty little habit of making junk food appear "healthier" than it truly is. "Fat free," "low sodium," "now with less sugar"…there is a seemingly endless series of gimmicks to describe the foods we buy. The reasons for this run deep into our product labelling policies, which are in serious need of revision (in my opinion). Until the glorious day when food producers are banned from touting junk as healthful, keep in mind that when it comes to food, a health claim does not mean that a food is healthy. Ideally, you should always be able to recognize the ingredients you are putting into your body. Read the ingredients label on the side of any packaged products you eat for the best information the package can provide to you. (Ingredients are listed by weight from heaviest to lightest.)

Let's review a few examples of what I like to call "healthy imposters":

Impostor #1: Chocolate-Hazelnut Spread

Chocolate-hazelnut spreads are often marketing as being "part of a well-balanced breakfast." Although these spreads probably aren't the worst thing you could be eating for breakfast, they're definitely not a good choice either. Their commercials focus on the hazelnuts and skim milk used to make the product but fail to tell you that the first ingredient on its label is actually sugar. Are hazelnuts or skim milk next on the list? Nope. Next on the ingredients list is modified palm oil. Although I do appreciate that most chocolate-hazelnut spreads only have about eight ingredients, real hazelnut spread only needs one: hazelnuts. And with a whopping 11 g of sugar and a measly 1 g of protein per tbsp, these spreads shouldn't be considered a healthy alternative to other nut butters, such as natural peanut butter, which, by comparison, has only 1 g of sugar (naturally occurring and not added) and 3 g of protein per tbsp. In the UK (where regulations about health claims are a bit stricter than in Canada), a TV ad for a popular chocolate-hazelnut spread was pulled by a regulatory agency after it concluded that the company's claims that it was a healthy breakfast choice were deemed false.[11] I'm not necessarily saying to never eat these sorts of spreads, but I am saying it's not a healthy breakfast choice.

Impostor #2: Highly Processed 100-Calorie "Snack Packs"

Just because something only has 100 calories, it doesn't make it a healthy choice. Yes, these snack packs are helpfully portioned for us. But the problem is that alongside the granola bars (which for the most part aren't very healthy either), these tiny bags of cookies and chips are now marketed as a healthy little treat to add in with your lunch. So now not only are you adding this into your lunch when you probably wouldn't ever have thought of packing its original version (snack mixes or cookies), but you're also bringing a little wafery version that doesn't even taste that great. Does anyone like the "thins" versions of anything? It's like eating cardboard full of either sugar or salt that provides no real nutrients along with the calories you're getting. Eating something that's actually filling like a piece of fruit will give you about the same calories, not leave you hungry 15 minutes later, and provide you with lots of other great vitamins and minerals...which leads me to our next impostor.

Impostor #3: Vitamin-Fortified Junk Food

This trend is the opposite of adding sugar to healthier foods (i.e., Impostor #1) but is becoming just as prevalent. The addition of vitamins or minerals to junk foods allows companies to make health claims to convince consumers the item is a good choice. Case in point: vitamin-enhanced water. It's not just water infused with vitamins, it's sugar-water infused with vitamins. Liquid calories are adding up in our diets like never before, so I'd prefer my water not to be adding to the trouble. Many other sugary sodas and juices are jumping on this bandwagon as well, so keep your common sense about you when buying items for specific vitamin claims.

These have been just a few examples of the countless healthy impostors out there lining our grocery store shelves. What's a consumer to do? First, remember that the more refined and packaged something becomes, the less likely it is to be healthy for you. Eat real food (i.e., comes from a garden or farm, is washed, then bought by you) as often as possible. For packaged items you can't live without—hey, I may be an idealist, but I'm still realistic—I can't emphasize enough the importance of reading the ingredients list. The nutrition facts label doesn't tell the whole story; for example, it does not distinguish between naturally occurring sugars and added sugars, so reading the ingredients label is arguably more important than anything else on the package. If you see sugar or salt within the first few ingredients, this is a red flag. Look beyond the front of the box (this is where companies put the things they *want* you to see) and turn it around. This is where you'll spot any information you should know that they fail to promote.

Final Note

As with any lifestyle change, it is important to consider the long-term implications of dietary changes that you choose to make. Fad diets often focus on severely restricting or entirely eliminating a certain food group or nutrient for a "quick fix." There are a few major problems with the approach of these restrictive diets: i) they can lead to nutrient deficiencies over time, ii) they leave us feeling deprived, and iii) they fail to address the root cause of our behaviours. Using the information and resources provided in this book (along with the inspiration of our incredible storytellers), identify and put into action just one thing you can change today to start eating for life. Eating well will help you to feel better in the short term and live healthier in the long term. Bon appétit!

Resources

Food Diary Template. This Canadian Obesity Network handout includes a detailed description, examples, and tips for completing a food diary:

www.obesitynetwork.ca/files/CON_HtKaFoodDiary_8.5x11.pdf

References

1. Bacon, L & L Aphramor. Weight Science: Evaluating the Evidence for a Paradigm Shift. *Nutr J.* 2011; 10:9. Available online at: www.ncbi.nlm.nih.gov/pmc/articles/PMC3041737/?tool=pubmed.

2. Kant, AK et al. Association of breakfast energy density with diet quality and body mass index in American adults: National Health and Nutrition Examination Surveys, 1999-2004. *Am J Clin Nutr.* 2008 Nov; 88(5): 1396-404.

3. Song, WO et al. Is consumption of breakfast associated with body mass index in US adults? *J Am Diet Assoc* 2005; 105: 1373-82.

4. Wyatt, HR et al. Long-term weight loss and breakfast in subjects in the National Weight Control Registry. *Obes Res* 2002; 10: 78-82.

5. Ma, Y et al. Association between eating patterns and obesity in a free-living US adult population. *Am J Epidemiol* 2003; 158: 85-92.

6. Health Canada. Drug Identification Number. Available online at: www.hc-sc.gc.ca/dhp-mps/prodpharma/activit/fs-fi/dinfs_fd-eng.php.

7. Health Canada. About Natural Health Product Regulation in Canada. Available online at: www.hc-sc.gc.ca/dhp-mps/prodnatur/about-apropos/index-eng.php.

8. Park, S et al. Multivitamin use and the risk of mortality and cancer incidence: the multiethnic cohort study. *Am J Epidemiol.* 2011 Apr 15;173(8): 906-14.

9. Huang, H et al. Multivitamin/mineral supplements and prevention of chronic disease. *Evid Rep Technol Assess* (Full Rep). 2006 May;(139): 1-117.

10. Health Canada. *Vitamin D and Calcium: Updated Dietary Reference Intakes.* November 2010. Available online at: www.hc-sc.gc.ca/fn-an/nutrition/vitamin/vita-d-eng.php.

11. BBC News. "Misleading" Nutella TV Ad Pulled. February 27, 2008. Available online at: http://news.bbc.co.uk/2/hi/uk_news/7266143.stm.

Chapter 14

Making the Best of the Rest of Your Life

"Life isn't about finding yourself. Life is about creating yourself" — George Bernard Shaw

We are given only one life in which to make an impact and to see and do what we want. When people on their deathbeds are asked if they have regrets, they do not tend to say, "I wish I was more active" or "I wish I ate healthier and got the proper amount of sleep." They may mention something about spending more time with their children or taking an adventure. We do the "healthy" things so that we can live our lives to the fullest.

When my friend Jane was sick with cancer, we would spend days in her basement dreaming about what the future held. At that point she could not do much else. It was honestly something I never put much thought into until then. My concerns up to that point were what classes I would take next semester and what boy was going to ask me to dance. We started dreaming about what we would like to accomplish, see, and do. We started a "bucket list" (or what I refer to as a "Life List" because it sounds more positive). The lists that we created included everything from going to Cuba (Jane's), going to an NHL playoff game (mine), learning three languages (Jane's), and bungee jumping (mine).

When she was losing hope, or feeling awful, we used to dream about what doing some of those things would be like. Jane had her wish granted by the Children's Wish Foundation and she chose to go to Cuba. During her treatment, when she was feeling well enough, she would go shopping for "Cuba clothes"—bathing suits, shorts, wraps, and sunglasses. She used to model them to keep her spirits up and keep focused on life after treatment.

When things took a turn for the worse and we knew she did not have much time left, Jane was moved to the palliative care part of the hospital. Her family and friends would wait in this small waiting room for when she was feeling well enough to see us. I remember spending hours in that waiting room and talking to friends who would stop by. Jane's family was in and out of her room and I have to admit I was in a daze just to get through. One time her father and I were sitting there, a seat between us, in silence. He said—and I will never forget this—"You cannot stop living, Lisa. Don't ever stop living. You are living for two now." I will never forget that moment. Although I may not have realized it then, it was a pivotal moment in my life: a game changer. At the time it felt like pressure I couldn't handle, and it would be a few years before I would truly understand.

Many of us strive to "live in the moment," but everything seems to creep in on this notion—work, deadlines, money, etc. I am very fortunate to have been able to work with cancer survivors while still in my 20s. These are individuals who value every moment, and it is contagious. Every time I get fixated on something, the survivors I work with always have insight or a story to shake me back into concentrating on what is important.

A couple of years after Jane passed, I was cleaning up (a rare event to say the least) and I found our list. I stopped cleaning immediately and I started to type it on my computer. Then I started adding to this list. I still missed Jane every day; she has inspired so much of what I did. The best way I could think of honouring Jane's memory was to become very serious about fulfilling this Life List that we had created together.

None of us know how many days we have left. It could be 60 years, 60 days, or 60 seconds. Alas, we cannot live in fear of this inevitability; we have to take it as a gift. It became my personal mission to add life into every day.

This list took on a bit of a life of its own. It surprised me how many adventures it has taken me on, how many people I have met, and how many experiences I would have never had if I had left my head down and chose not to take action.

I am very careful with my money, unless it comes to the list. I believe that Life List items are the reason credit cards exist. (Don't tell my financial advisor I said that.) So far I have gone bungee jumping, shaved my head for cancer, run a marathon in Paris, met Richard Simmons (okay that wasn't on the list, but it was pretty cool), gone skydiving, helped build a house with Habitat for Humanity, learned to rock climb, got three tattoos, saw a play on Broadway, and wrote a book...just to name a few.

It isn't just crossing off the things off the list that makes this concept so important, it is the adventures that happen along the way. It is the friendships you make, the people who inspire you, and who you inspire. Do not wait until you are faced with death to begin living. Actually, don't wait another second. I encourage you—no, I *challenge* you—to think about what you want to accomplish with your life. In our goal setting chapter, we talked about setting "realistic" goals. This is very true for health behaviours, but when it comes to your life, dream big. Have fun thinking about how to make the impossible possible and just go for it.

"A journey of a thousand miles begins with a single step."
— Lao Tzu

Grab a pen, paper, your phone, or computer and start dreaming. I suggest discussing these ideas with others; you may come up with more than you thought. Take care of your body to get you through the list.

"To live is the rarest thing in the world. Most people exist, that is all." — Oscar Wilde

For some ideas, take a look at our lists:

Lisa's Bucket List

1. ~~Skydive~~
2. Visit each continent
3. Be in a commercial
4. Adopt a child
5. ~~Shave head for cancer~~
6. Take a road trip across Canada
7. Go to an NHL playoff game
8. ~~Go to a Broadway musical...on Broadway~~
9. ~~Bungee jump~~
10. Go to Cuba and write my name in the sand
11. Snowboard at Whistler
12. ~~Learn to surf~~
13. Own a dog
14. ~~Get an article published~~
15. ~~Get my X ring (The graduation ring from St. Francis Xavier University)~~
16. Become a doctor (PhD style)
17. Witness an eclipse
18. Meet someone famous
19. ~~Meet someone with the same name as me~~
20. Learn about photography
21. Run a marathon
22. ~~Help build a house~~
23. Participate in a triathlon
24. Attend the Olympics
25. Attend a football game in Europe
26. Teach someone to read

27. Get my future told by a psychic
28. Drink a vintage wine
29. Bike the Cabot Trail
30. ~~Rock climb~~
31. Ride a horse
32. ~~Go fishing~~
33. Learn a third language
34. Teach yoga or dance
35. Learn martial arts
36. See the Great Pyramid of Giza
37. Bike across a country (country to be determined)
38. Skate on the Ottawa Canal
39. Skinny-dip
40. Coach a winning soccer and hockey team
41. Own a house
42. Play beach soccer
43. See the northern lights
44. Try hand gliding
45. Take a hot-air balloon ride
46. Ride a motorcycle
47. Attempt drunk bowling
48. Drive a Mercedes-Benz or BMW worth more than $40,000 (preferably owned by me)
49. ~~Snorkel the Great Barrier Reef~~
50. ~~Write a book~~
51. Swim with dolphins
52. Win an award
53. Learn to play guitar
54. Catch a fish with my bare hands
55. Leave my mark with graffiti
56. Get a piece of art into an exhibit
57. Ride the world's fastest and tallest roller coasters
58. Crowd-surf

59. Stay in the best suite at a four-star hotel
60. Design my own cocktail
61. Fly first class on an airplane
62. Throw a dart onto the map and travel where it lands
63. Attend a film premiere
64. Milk a cow
65. Write my name over a star on the Walk of Fame
66. Experience a sunset and sunrise on the same night
67. Make a purchase I cannot afford
68. Give someone a heartfelt surprise
69. Invent a game or app
70. Make the front page of a newspaper
71. Drive a car at top speed
72. Save someone's life
73. Have enough money to do everything on this list
74. Create a legacy
75. Get three tattoos
76. Learn astrology
77. Spend Christmas on a beach
78. Get banned from a bar or pub
79. Learn to salsa dance
80. Eat at Serendipity, NYC
81. Get married unusually
82. Complete Monopoly pub crawl in London
83. Get something named after me
84. Be an extra in a film
85. Tag along for a protest
86. Go to the horse, dog, or camel races
87. Laugh so hard I cry
88. Be in two places at once
89. Walk on water

90. Give a keynote address
91. Be in Women's Health magazine
92. Climb Mt. Everest or Mt. Kilimanjaro
93. Dress up and go to Super Bowl
94. Write a children's book
95 Go to Beerfest
96. Go on tour of the Lindt chocolate factory
97. Get drunk with Paul and Cheryl Bélanger
98. Go to a talk show filming
99. Spend St. Paddy's day in Ireland
100. Own a pair of Manolo Blahnik or Jimmy
     Choo shoes

.

Sarah's Bucket List

1. ~~Write a book~~
2. Tour Europe
3. Run my own business
4. Half-marathon PB under 1:50
5. Acquire my Red Seal chef certification
6. ~~Take a bike tour through wine country~~
7. Visit every Canadian province and territory
8. Go deep-sea fishing
9. Ride in a helicopter
10. Mush a dogsled
11. Visit my dad's birth town in England
12. Visit my mom's father's gravesite in Germany
13. Take singing lessons
14. Compose a song
15. ~~Snorkel or scuba dive in underwater caves~~
16. Go hiking in a rainforest
17. Visit the seven wonders of the world
18. Visit Disney World

19. Learn to garden
20. Start a community garden project
21. Provide nutrition or medical aid in a developing country
22. Ride in a hot air balloon
23. Participate in a flash mob
24. Own a waterfront cottage
25. See a World Series Championship baseball game
26. Become a wine connoisseur
27. Go one month without buying anything for myself (except food)
28. Learn how to make chocolates
29. ~~Drink in an Irish Pub (in Ireland)~~
30. Be an extra in a feature film or television show
31. Go cycling in Spain
32. Watch the Tour de France in person
33. Learn to make my own clothing
34. Host an out-of-country exchange student
35. Swim in the Dead Sea

For more inspiration and to create your own Life List, check out *www.mylifelist.org*. What does your list look like? What will your story be? What is your legacy? Whatever it is, we encourage you to start today. *This* is the rest of your life. Taking care of your body and health will take you beyond what you ever thought possible. We genuinely hope that the stories of our contributors have inspired you as much as they have us and that the additional information we have provided is useful in harnessing your motivation to start living a healthier and more fulfilling life.

We tend to set limits for ourselves, but when we accept that there are no boundaries, limits no longer exist. Greatness is achieved.

Afterword

By Timothy Caulfield

A recent paper in the *New England Journal of Medicine* enumerated the ways in which most of us will die. It highlighted that a profound shift has occurred over the past 100 years. In 1900 the biggest threats to our mortality were things like pneumonia, tuberculosis, and gastrointestinal infection—all conditions to which both public health policy (e.g., sanitation systems) and biomedical science (e.g., antibiotics) responded to with notable success. Today, especially in the developed countries, the biggest killers are, by far, cancer and heart disease. And as in the past, success in combating these diseases will require a combination of public health and biomedical innovation.

But the challenge is great. Cancer, for example, is proving to be a phenomenally complex disease. And the public health interventions that are most needed—more nutritious diets, less smoking, a reduction in the rates of obesity, and an increase in physical activity—all require behaviour change. Sadly, experience and research tell us that we humans do not like to change our behaviour, particularly in the direction of less food and more activity.

To make matters worse, popular culture is awash in misinformation about nutrition and exercise. Indeed, there is likely more information in circulation about trendy (and largely useless) diets and exercise routines than the simple truths about the basic elements of a healthy lifestyle. It should be no surprise that few

Canadians eat a balanced diet, exercise enough, or even know how many calories they eat or should eat.

Inspire Me Well is aimed at the heart of the behaviour change dilemma. Early in the book the authors remind us that a large portion of our health is the result of is "the sum of many small choices we make daily." The book then provides a unique and effective mix of health research, practical advice, and personal (and often very moving) stories that are designed to, yep, inspire us well. The book covers everything from diet to exercise to when to go to the doctor. And it notes the importance of the social, and often under-emphasized, aspects of a healthy lifestyle, including parental and family support and the reduction of stress.

Too often we, as a society, seem fixated on high-tech and scientifically complex approaches to health issues. But, as noted by the authors of the NEJM paper, "[d]iseases can never be reduced to molecular pathways, mere technical problems requiring treatments or cures."[1] It is also a social phenomenon that requires a social response. It requires the promotion of a healthy lifestyle, at both the level of the individual and the population. As this book suggests, future health policy needs to place a greater emphasis on the creation of a society where healthy decisions are easier to make. This will mean, among other things, greater access to nutritious food options, education programs that provide appropriate life skills, and the creation of an environment that encourages and promotes physical activity.

While this kind of shift will always require a careful balancing between the protection of individual liberties (if people want to live like sloths, can we stop them?) and potentially coercive health policy, encouraging (or, at least, *inspiring*) healthy decisions can never be a bad idea!

Reference

1. Jones, DS, SH Podolsky, & JA Greene. The Burden of Disease and the Changing Task of Medicine. *N Engl J Med* 2012; 366: 2333–38.

Timothy Caulfield is a Canada Research Chair in Health Law and Policy and a Professor in the Faculty of Law and the School of Public Health at the University of Alberta. He is also the Research Director of the Health Law and Science Policy Group (HeaLS). Over the past several years, he has been involved in a variety of interdisciplinary research endeavours that have allowed him to publish over 250 articles and book chapters. He has won numerous academic awards, publishes frequently in the popular press, has been involved with a number of national and international policy and research ethics committees, and is the author of the bestselling book The Cure for Everything: Untangling the Twisted Messages about Health, Fitness and Happiness *(Penguin Canada). He is a Fellow of the Royal Society of Canada and the Canadian Academy of Health Sciences.*

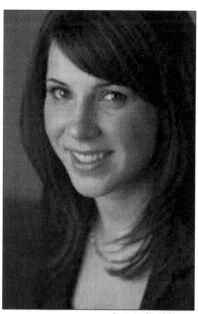
Photo by Cindy Gannon

Lisa Bélanger is the owner of Exceed Wellness, a PhD candidate at the University of Alberta, and a certified exercise physiologist from the Canadian Society of Exercise Physiology. Lisa received her undergraduate degree in Human Kinetics and Psychology with honours from St. Francis Xavier University. It was there she began to use her passion for physical activity to inspire others and started personal training. She completed her Masters of Science in Physical Education and Recreation from the University of Alberta; her research focused on the impact physical activity can have on cancer survivors. This research is now being continued into her PhD. She has experience with elite athletes, as well as clients interested in weight loss, building muscle mass, and general fitness. Lisa was one of *Edmontonian*'s Top 20 under 30 in 2010 and was the winner of the YMCA Woman of Influence—Local Hero Award.

@lisabelanger13
lisa@exceedwellness.ca

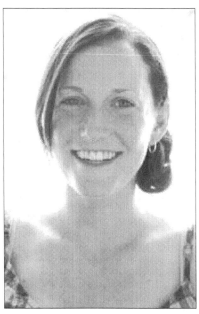
Photo by Jessica Fern Facette

Sarah O'Hara is a Registered Dietitian who is passionate about chronic disease prevention and management through lifestyle modification. She completed her nutrition studies at the University of Alberta with an Integrated Dietetic Internship Program. Prior to her pursuit of dietetics, Sarah received a Bachelor of Science majoring in Biology and Psychology from the University of New Brunswick and also holds a Diploma in University Teaching (an Adult Education program) from the same institution. Sarah's goal is to provide highly personalized nutrition and lifestyle counseling by allowing each of her clients to find inspiration for lifelong healthy living within their resources.

@SarahFOHara
info@inspiremewell.com

19822239R00114

Made in the USA
Lexington, KY
08 January 2013